Stéphane Fargeon MBOUNA MASSIN
Bernadette NGO NONGA
Georges BWELLE

Chest trauma in Africa

Stéphane Fargeon MBOUNA MASSIN
Bernadette NGO NONGA
Georges BWELLE

Chest trauma in Africa

Current state of thoracic trauma from 2016 to 2020 in Cameroon

ScienciaScripts

Imprint
Any brand names and product names mentioned in this book are subject to trademark, brand or patent protection and are trademarks or registered trademarks of their respective holders. The use of brand names, product names, common names, trade names, product descriptions etc. even without a particular marking in this work is in no way to be construed to mean that such names may be regarded as unrestricted in respect of trademark and brand protection legislation and could thus be used by anyone.

Cover image: www.ingimage.com

This book is a translation from the original published under ISBN 978-620-6-70321-1.

Publisher:
Sciencia Scripts
is a trademark of
Dodo Books Indian Ocean Ltd. and OmniScriptum S.R.L publishing group

120 High Road, East Finchley, London, N2 9ED, United Kingdom
Str. Armeneasca 28/1, office 1, Chisinau MD-2012, Republic of Moldova, Europe
Printed at: see last page
ISBN: 978-620-8-30312-9

Contents

DEDICATION

To my late grandmother,

KEMEGNI Elise

ACKNOWLEDGEMENTS

I would like to express my sincere thanks:

> To the Lord **Jesus Christ**, without whom I would not be of this world today.

> To the **promoter** and **director** of the Institut Supërieur de Technologie Mëdicale

> To **Prof. NGO NONGA Bernadette**, my тёrе, my lifelong master, the best surgeon I know and my tlrese director. You have been my mentor since the very beginning of my clinical aniK'es. Thank you very much. May God bless you.

> To **Dr. BWELLE Motto Georges**, my co-director, who has followed this work from beginning to end and is the best anatomy teacher I know. Thank you very much. May God bless you.

> To **Dr. BITANG A MAFOK Louis**, my second co-director, for your guidance and direction. Thank you very much. May God bless you.

> To all the administrative and teaching staff of the Institut Supërieur de Technologie Mëdicale

> To my grandmother, the late mother **KEMEGNI Elise**, who paid my first-year tuition fees when my parents didn't have a penny. So I was able to secure my place at ISTM.

> To **ONGBENOK Florence** and to **MBOUNA Frederic**, my parents, who worked so hard first to bring me up and then to enable me to go to school to learn this beautiful trade. I am very grateful to you all.

> To **NOUMEYI MAFO Sanita**, the love of my life and the woman of my dreams, who has supported me enormously during this year of preparation for my tlK'se. My princess, I love you. You are the best.

> To **MBOUNA Ghislaine Diane**, my great-sister, for all her support. May God bën bless you abundantly with all kinds of graces.

> To **Dr. BALKISSOU Dodo**, my clinical sëmiology teacher. You believed in my abilities, even though I doubted that I would ever be able to make a good medical observation. Thank you very much. May God bless you.

> To all my internship supervisors at CHUY, HCY and HGY who regu and йзтё me during the acadëmiques internships.

> To **Dr. EDINGA Elodie**, for all your encouragement. May God bless you.

> To **Dr. BANGA**, for his advice in drafting my investigation form. May God bless you.

> To the staff and directors of the Ad-Luchem Banka-Bafang hospital and the Sangmëlima district hospital, where I did my integrated medicine course.

> To **Joyce Meyer**, my Bible teacher and the one who helped me through the wounds of my past.

> To the Groupe Biblique des Eteves et Etudiants du Cameroun (GBEEC) for all your teachings on issues relating to fellowship.

> To all the evangelisation team (EVA32) in which I took my first steps in the Christian faith.

> To you, the **Superstudents**, the 8th graduating class of the Institut Superieur de Technologie Medicale, thank you for sharing your thoughts and experiences.

> Many thanks and blessings to all those who have contributed to this work, either directly or indirectly.

HIPPOCRATIC OATH

Adoptë par la 2eme assemble дёпёrale de l'Association Mëdicale Mondiale, Geneve (Suisse), septembre 1948, et amendë par la 22eme assembke тёёкяк mondiale, Sydney, Australia, August 1968, and the 35th World Assembke Мёёкяк, Venice, Italy, October 1983, and the 46th World Assembkc Мёёкяк, Stockholm, Sweden, September 1994, and rëvisë by the 170th Council Session, Divonne-les-Bains, France, May 2005, and by the 173rd Council Session, Divonne-les-Bains, France, May 2006 and amendë by the 68th Gerarale Assembke de l'Association Medicale Mondiale in October 2017.

As a member of the medical profession

I solemnly undertake to devote my life to the service of humanity; I will consider the health and well-being of my patient as my priority;

I will respect my patient's autonomy and dignity;

I will ensure absolute respect for human life;

I will not allow considerations of age, illness or disability, creed, ethnic origin, gender, nationality, political affiliation, race, sexual orientation, social status or any other factor to come between my duty and my patient;

I will respect the secrets entrusted to me, even after the death of my patient;

I will practise my profession with conscience and dignity, in accordance with good medical practice;

I will perpetuate the honour and noble traditions of the medical profession;

I will show my teachers, colleagues and students the respect and recognition they deserve;

I will share my medical knowledge for the benefit of patients and the advancement of healthcare

I will look after my own health and wellbeing and will continue my training so that I can provide irreproachable care;

I will not use my medical knowledge to infringe human rights and civil liberties, even under duress;

I make these promises on my honour, solemnly and freely

SUMMARY

Background: Thoracic trauma is the second leading cause of death Hëc a trauma in the world. Their incidence is constantly increasing in Sub-Saharan Africa. The lesions are often insidious and unrecognised. Nevertheless, prompt treatment is essential. The aim of this study was therefore to describe the management of thoracic trauma in two referral hospitals in Yaounde.

Methodology: We conducted a cross-sectional study with retrospective data collection from 1er January 2016 to 31 December 2020 at the Yaounde University Hospital and the Yaounde Emergency Centre. The records of 358 patients admitted for thoracic trauma who met the inclusion criteria were recorded in a database created using CsPro 7.6.0 software. It was then analysed using SPSS Statistics 23 software. The results were presented in the form of tables and figures in MS Word and Excel 2019.

Results: The majority of victims were men aged between 16 and 44, with a sex ratio of 5H/1F. The median age was 30 (1-96) years. The frequency of thoracic trauma was 16.5%. One in three patients was arrreë less than one hour after l'accident. Firm trauma (89%) was predominant. Traffic accidents (67.5%) and stabbings (88%) were the two main causes of firm and penetrating trauma respectively. Pulmonary contusion (65.3%) was the most frequent lesion. Cranioencephalic trauma (56.6%) was the main associated lesion. Management modalities were conservative treatment alone (69.9%), pleural drainage associated with conservative treatment (12.3%) and thoracotomy (7.3%). One patient in three developed complications, the main one being acute respiratory distress syndrome. The overall mortality rate was 13.6%.

Conclusion: The means of treatment available in our environment make it possible to achieve a morbidity and mortality similar to that found in the West. Prompt treatment will optimise patient care.

Key words : Thoracic trauma; Management; Current situation; Cameroon

I-INTROD UCTION

The World Health Organisation (WHO) defines trauma as sudden bodily injury resulting from acute exposure to external energy (mechanical, thermal, electrical, chemical or radiant) at a level that exceeds physiological tolerance [1]. Chest trauma refers to physical injury to the chest wall and/or its container caused by an external agent [1]. The United States Department of Veterans Affairs defines polytrauma as the presence of at least one lesion on at least two organs belonging to two different systems, one of which may be life-threatening in the short or long term, and which may result in physical, cognitive or psychosocial dysfunction and functional disability [2]. Thoracic injuries are classified into closed and penetrating injuries [3]. Thoracic lesions are particularly difficult to treat and can rapidly form fatal vicious circles [3]. In addition, thoracic trauma is very frequently found in the context of polytrauma [4].

Thoracic trauma is a major public health problem [5]. According to the WHO, they are responsible for the deaths of around one million people each year, making them the second leading cause of death in trauma [5]. Their incidence is increasing by an average of five per cent a year, with a clear predominance in Africa [5]. In Germany, they are the leading cause of death in trauma emergencies [6]. Africa accounts for ninety per cent of global trauma deaths [7]. Furthermore, in sub-Saharan Africa, the annual cost of treating these injuries is ninety billion US dollars, or two per cent of gross domestic product [8]. In South Africa, one in three trauma patients admitted to emergency departments dies as a result of a thoracic injury [9]. In Cameroon, this mortality rate is estimated at ten per cent by the WHO [10]. In addition, less than twenty per cent of healthcare staff in district hospitals in the Centre region state that they are qualified to manage patients with chest trauma [11].

Traffic accidents and stabbings are the main causes of firm and penetrating injuries respectively worldwide [12]. However, in the United States and in war zones, ballistic trauma is the leading cause of penetrating injury [13,14]. In Cameroon, road traffic accidents and stabbings are incriminated in the occurrence of most thoracic injuries, and two-thirds of these lesions are closed [15]. The diagnosis of thoracic lesions requires careful clinical examination and often necessitates the performance of paraclinical examinations [16]. Standard radiography and, to a lesser extent, thoracic ultrasound are generally the only two imaging tests available in our context [17].

Management of victims of thoracic trauma begins at the scene of the incident with first aid, and should continue during transport to the emergency department and then, if necessary, to the operating theatre or intensive care unit [18]. Lesions are treated conservatively or surgically [18]. The indications for thoracic drainage are the subject of much controversy [18]. The choice of treatment modality depends on the patient's hemodynamic state, the nature of the lesion and the more or less long-term prognosis [18]. Worldwide, more than three-quarters of patients receive conservative treatment, sometimes combined with thoracic drainage [18]. In Cameroon, at the Yaounde General Hospital in 2003, more than eight out of ten patients received conservative treatment combined with thoracic drainage, and one out of ten received thoracotomy [19].

Some ten years later, it seemed appropriate to us to conduct a study with the aim of taking stock of the management of thoracic trauma in two referral hospitals in Yaounde, in order to identify data that could be used in the development of a national protocol for the management of these lesions.

II-RESEARCH QUESTION

Research question

What are the management modalities for thoracic trauma usedëes at the Yaounde Hospital and University Centre and the Yaounde Emergency Centre from 1er January 2016 to 31 December 2020?

Research hypothesis

The methods used to treat thoracic trauma between 1er January 2016 and 31 December 2020 at the Yaounde University Hospital and the Yaounde Emergency Centre are different from those used in the past.

III-OBJECTIVES

1-General objective

To help optimise the management of thoracic trauma victims in our context.

2-Specific objectives

i-Define the sociodëmographic, clinical and paraclinical profile of these patients.

2-Determine the annual frequency of thoracic trauma in emergency departments.

3-Describe the different ways of managing lesions and the indications for thoracotomy.

4-Picture the complications and vital prognosis of patients suffering chest trauma.

IV-LITERATURE REVIEW

A. Review of knowledge

IV.1 Anatomical and physiological background

IV.1.1 Anatomical background [22,23].

IV.1.1.1 Chest wall anatomy

The thorax is the body cavity, surrounded by the bony rib cage, which contains the hollow cavity and lungs, the large vessels of the hollow cavity, the resophagus, the trachea, the thoracic duct and the autonomic innervation of these structures. The lower limit of the thoracic cavity is the diaphragm, which separates the thoracic and abdominal cavities. Superiorly, the thorax communicates with the root of the neck and the upper limb. The thorax is covered by skin and superficial fascia containing breast tissue.

The curved shape of the ribcage provides remarkable rigidity, given the lightness of its contents, enabling it to :

> Protect vital internal thoracic and abdominal organs from external forces.

> Resist the negative (sub-atmospheric) internal pressures generated by the elastic recoil of the lungs and inspiratory movements.

> Support the weight of your upper limbs.

> Serve as the anchor point for numerous muscles which, by moving, maintain the position of the upper limbs in relation to the trunk, as well as the insertion points for certain muscles in the abdomen, neck and back, and are involved in breathing.

IV.1.1.1.1 Chest wall skeleton

There are three types of ratings:

- **True ribs** or vertebro-costals (from the 1ere to the 7eme ribs): they are attached directly to the sternum by their own costal cartilage.
- **False** or vertebrochondral **ribs** (from the 8eme to the 10eme ribs): their cartilages are connected to the overlying costal cartilage. Their connection with the sternum is indirect.
- **Floating** or vertebral **ribs** (11eme and 12eme ribs): the rudimentary cartilages of these ribs do not connect indirectly with the sternum; instead, they terminate in the posterior abdominal musculature.

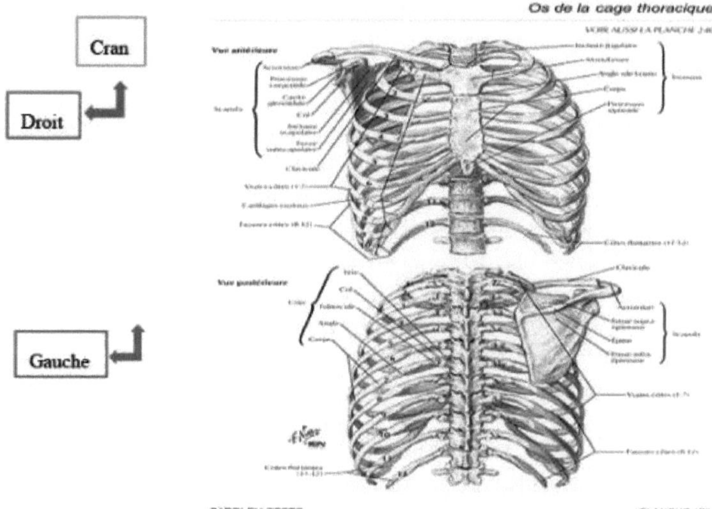

Figure 1. Bone architecture of the thorax [23].

IV.1.1.1.2 Chest wall muscles

There are: in front, the pectoralis major, pectoralis minor, subclavian and dentalis anterior muscles, the ëlëvator muscles of the ribs, the intercostals, subcostals and transverse thoracic muscle, the antërolatëral abdominal muscles in front; the dorsalis major, dentalis major and dentalis minor postëriere; the sternocleidomastoid and scalene muscles above. The scalene muscles, which descend to the first and second ribs.

IV.1.1.1.3 Vascularisation and innervation of the chest wall

> Arterial vascularisation

The arterial supply to the chest wall arises from :

- Thoracic aorta: posterior intercostal and subcostal arteries.
- Subclavian arteries: the internal thoracic and upper intercostal arteries
- Axillary artery: the superior and lateral thoracic arteries.

> Venous vascularisation

The intercostal veins are satellites of the arteries draining respectively :

- Most of the postëterior intercostal veins drain into the azygos/hemi-azygos venous system.
- The anterior intercostal veins drain into the internal thoracic veins.
- **Innervation of the chest wall**

The anterior branches of the T1 to T11 nerves form the intercostal nerves, which run along the length of the intercostal spaces. The anterior branch of the T12 nerve, which runs below the 12eme rib, is the subcostal nerve. The posterior branches of the thoracic spinal nerves pass posteriorly, innervating the joints, muscles and skin of the back in the thoracic region.

IV.1.1.2 Anatomy of the diaphragm

The diaphragm is a musculo-tendinous partition serving as an interface between the thorax and the abdomen. The muscle fibres of the diaphragm arise radially from the edges

of the lower thoracic opening and converge towards a large central tendon. Because of the obiquity of the lower thoracic opening, the posterior insertions of the diaphragm are inferior to the anterior insertions. The right dome is higher than the left.
In its upper part, it is vascularised by the pericardo-phrenic and musculo-phrenic arteries, branches of the internal thoracic artery. The upper phrenic arteries arise directly from the lower part of the thoracic aorta, and from small branches of the intercostal arteries. The inferior phrenic arteries are the largest arteries supplying the diaphragm and arise from the abdominal aorta. Venous drainage of the diaphragm is via the brachiocephalic veins, the system of azygos veins, the left supra-renal vein and the inferior vena cava. It is innervated by the phrenic nerves (C3 to C5).

IV.1.1.3 The mediastinum

The mediastinum extends from the sternum at the front to the thoracic spine at the back, and from the upper orifice to the lower orifice of the thorax. It is bordered on each side by the pleuropulmonary regions.

IV.1.1.3.1 The superior mediastinum

It meets the sternal manubrium at the front and contains: the resophagus, the trachea, the aortic arch and its branches, the brachio-cephalic venous trunks, the thoracic duct, the upper half of the superior vena cava, the thymus or its remnants, the right and left phrenic, pneumogastric, cardiac and left recurrent nerves, the arterial ligament, the paratracheal and superior tracheobronchial lymph nodes and the arch of the azygos.

IV.1.1.3.2 The anterior mediastinum

Very narrow, it meets the sternal body at the front and the anterior face of the pericardium at the back. It contains: the internal thoracic vessels and the parasternal and pre-pericardial lymph nodes.

IV.1.1.3.3 The middle mediastinum

The middle mediastinum contains: the pericardial sac and its contents, the pulmonary vessels, the latëro-pericardial and inferior tracheo-bronchial lymph nodes.

IV.1.1.3.4 Posterior mediastinum

The posterior mediastinum contains: the descending thoracic aorta, the thoracic resophagus, the thoracic duct, the azygos and hemi-azygos veins, the pneumogastric and splanchnic nerves, the juxta-resophageal, prevertebral and superior phrenic pulmonary ganglia.

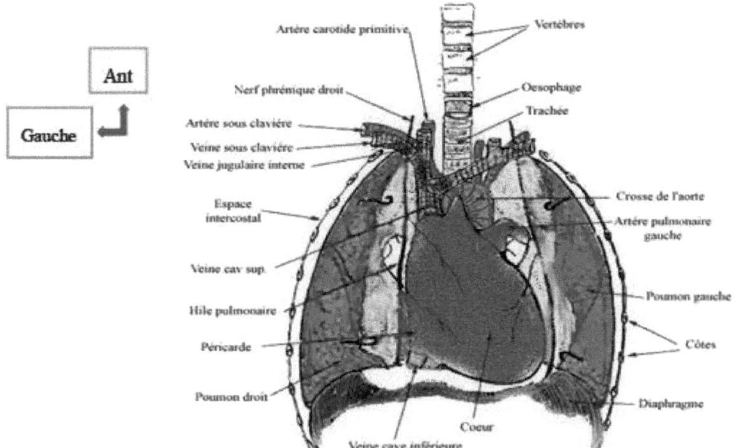

Figure 2. Superior view of the middle mediastinum [23].

IV.1.1.4 Anatomy of the levator vein

The vein that lines the wall of the thoracic cavity is called the parietal vein; it is rëAëeЫ1 in the mediastinum around the pedicle, where it is continuous with the visceral vein that lines the surface of the lungs. The space between the visceral pleura lining the walls of the thoracic cavity is normally virtual.

IV.1.1.4.1 The parietal vein

> Positioning and ratios :

- The parietal pleura rests on the deep surface of the thoracic wall via a layer of cellulo-fatty tissue: the subpleural fascia or endothoracic fascia. This avascular endothoracic fascia forms a cleavage plane known as the extrapleural plane, which can be used to free the levator and the lung when the levator is completely fused.
- On the deep surface of the ribs and intercostal spaces, the endothoracic fascia is thick, dense and well individualised.
- In front, behind the sternum, and behind at the level of the latero-vertebral grooves, it is extremely thin and sends a few fibrous tracts to the front of the thoracic spine.
- Below, at the level of the diaphragm, it is almost non-existent and the parietal membrane adheres strongly to the muscle. There is no cleavage plane between the levator and the diaphragm.
- Internally, it continues with the cellular tissue of the mediastinum.

At the top, it densifies considerably above the upper orifice of the thorax and forms Bourgery's cervico-thoracic diaphragm "Membrana Supra Pleuralis".

> Vascularisation and innervation :

The parietal vein contains the arterial and venous lymphatic vessels and the neighbouring nerves: internal thoracic and intercostal arteries. The corresponding veins drain into the inferior vena cava and the nerve branches come from the intercostal nerves, phrenic nerves and sympathetic trunks.

IV.1.1.4.2 The visceral vein

> Positioning and relationships :

It covers the entire surface of the lung, with the exception of part of the mediastinal side, where it reflects at the level of the hilum onto the elements of the pulmonary pedicle to become the parietal levator. This line of reflection continues below the hilum to form the triangular ligament. The levator also lines the bottom of the pulmonary scissures that separate the different lobes of the lung. The viscëral pleura is joined to the lung parenchyma by a thin layer of sub pleural cellular tissue which continues inside the parenchyma to form the interstitium of the lung.

> Vascularisation and innervation :

Branches of the bronchial arteries, venous drainage dependent on the pulmonary veins. The lymphatics and nerves are those of the lung.

IV.1.2 Physiological background [24]

IV.1.2.1 Breathing function

The respiratory muscles are innervated by nerves of bulbar and cervical origin, which constitute the pathways of neurons with inspiratory and expiratory activity, thus forming the generator or respiratory centre.

IV.1.2.2 Metabolic function

> Acid-base balance

> Regulation of systemic blood pressure by synthesis of angiotensin I to angiotensin II converting enzyme.

> Surfactant production by type II pneumocytes

IV.1.2.3 Thermolytic function

Inhaled air is generally colder and drier than exhaled air. By cooling and desiccating the alveolar gas during exhalation, the airways can recover some of the heat and moisture lost during inspiration.

IV.1.2.4 Purification and immune defence functions

There are three types of alveolar defence:

> The cells of the immune system are essentially macrophages, whose main role is to ensure phagocytosis.

> Alveolar ventilation depends on maintaining alveolar stability. A liquid film that moistens the alveolar wall, supplied by transudation from the capillaries, contributes to alveolar equilibrium.

> Lymphatic drainage contributes to the purification of particles.

IV.1.2.5 Plevre functions

The parietal plevre has a clë role in the formation and resorption of fluids and protëines. Liquid formation is 0.15 ml/kg/hr. This fluid contains surfactant-lamellar mokcules that promote sliding of the pleural sheets in contact.

IV.2 Pathophysiology [25]

In the event of thoracic trauma, there may initially be a dual respiratory and hëmodynamic failure, the genesis of which is multifactorial.

IV.2.1. Respiratory distress

It results from damage to ventilatory mechanics and/or inadequate ventilation/perfusion. Damage to the chest wall muscles of the costal gril and/or the diaphragm alters ventilatory mechanics, resulting in a^olar hypoventilation. This phënomëne is aggravated in the event of loss of pleural vacuum by the formation of a ëpanchement aërique ou liquidien qui dësolidarise le poumon de la paroi thoracique et du diaphragme dont les mouvements ne sont plus transmis lui.

IV.2.2. Cardiac and circulatory distress

This distress may be due to :

> Cardiogenic shock: myocardial contusion with valvular ksion, cardiac tamponade, compressive hëmopneumothorax which constitute an obstacle to filling.

> Hypovotemic shock due to extëriorised or non-extëriorised hëmorrhage (rupture of the aorta, supra-aortic vessels, massive hëmothorax).

> Mëdullary lesions of the dorsal spine, responsible for vasoplegia by sympathetic blockade which majors the hëmodynamic disorders.

IV.3 Lesion mechanisms [29].

There is no absolute paralklism between parietal and endothoracic ksions especially in young adults due to the flexibility of the skeleton.

> **Direct shock is the** most frequent mechanism. The gravitë is Hëc to the kinetic energy of the vulnerable agent striking the thorax. At the siëge of impact, we can observe:

❖ Compression or crushing injuries with parietal damage in the foreground (rib fractures, sternum fractures, costal flap, rupture of the diaphragm and fracture of the dorsal spine). In the background, there are pulmonary and/or cardiac contusions and tears of the lower thoracic aorta.

❖ Direct impact lesions with a closed glottis, the consëquences of which are due to tracheobronchial hyperpressure.

> **Lesions caused by deceleration**: intrathoracic lesions differ according to the amount of kinetic energy:

❖ Lesions caused by shearing or tearing: rupture of the aortic isthmus, thrombosis of the brachio-cephalic trunk, tracheo-bronchial rupture, rupture of the resophagus, thoracic duct wound.

❖ Impingement lesions such as pulmonary contusion due to impingement on the costal grill and myocardial contusion due to crushing of the heart muscle on the posterior wall of the sternum.

> **Blast damage** (shockwave or blast)

❖ The primary lesions by abdominal compression with ascension of the diaphragm and projection of the lung against the thoracic wall Hëc to the variation in the velocity of propagation of the wave, presenting a picture of alveolo-venous fistula with risk of gas embolism.

❖ Secondary lesions caused by the environment being projected onto the victim: direct impact.

❖ Tertiary lesions caused by the victim being thrown against his environment: dëcëlëration.

IV.4 Clinical forms [30-45]

IV.4.1 Rib fractures [30,31].

Rib fractures are an important part of thoracic trauma. The exact incidence is unknown. In a cohort of thoracic trauma patients admitted to intensive care, unilateral rib fractures were ëΓë found in 60% of cases. The number of fractured ribs dëpended on the mëcanism [30]. The energy required to induce a rib fracture is inversely proportional to the victim's age. Fracture of the first rib is rare. This fracture is a marker of severity [30]. An arterial anomaly is found in 14% of patients with this fracture [31]. Fractures of the last rib are associated with abdominal lesions.

IV.4.2 Costal flap [32].

A rib flap occurs when a segment of the chest wall becomes detached from the rest of the wall. This requires multiple fractures of adjacent ribs at multiple sites on the same side and separation of a segment causing paradoxical movement. This increases the work of breathing and the pain. The costal flap is accompanied by pulmonary contusion and possibly a hemopneumothorax.

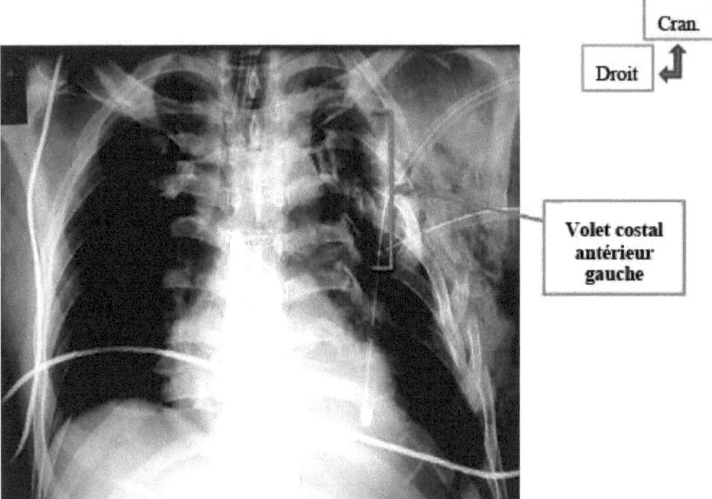

Figure 3. Left costal flap [25]

IV.4.3 Sternal fractures [33].

Sternal fractures are observed in road accident victims who suffer an impact with the steering wheel. Airbags currently protect against this type of lesion. Other causes are falls or direct blows. Rib fractures, myocardial contusions and pulmonary contusions are associated in 30% of cases.

IV.4.4 Diaphragmatic ruptures and hernias [34-36].

The right hdmi-diaphragm is ruptured in 15-20% of cases and the left in 70-80%. Clinically, patients may be asymptomatic. Dyspnea, chest pain, abdominal pain and vomiting may occur. Decreased vësicular murmur is the first finding. Bowel sounds in the chest are pathognomonic of intestinal hernias. The chest X-ray should be rëpëtëe. A thoraco-abdominal ëchography provides valuable information. Computed tomography is used secondarily. Retro-costo-xiphoid or Morgagni-Larrey hernias are more common in adults than cupola or Bochdalek hernias. They are sometimes responsible for acute abdomen. Diagnosis is based on chest X-ray and CT scan.
with barytëe opacification.

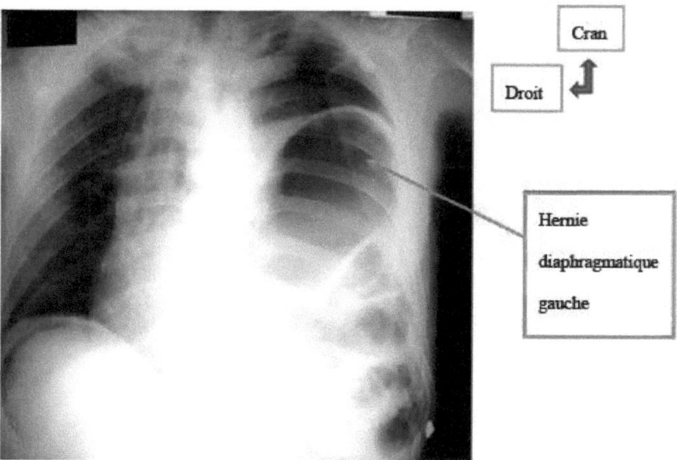

Figure 4: Strong suspicion of a ruptured left diaphragmatic cupola and probable associated hernia [25].

IV.4.5 Hemothorax [37]

I. Hemothorax is a collection of blood in the space between the chest wall and the lung, known as the pleural cavity. It is secondary to rib fractures, vertebral fractures or laceration of the lung. The clinical picture can be summed up as hypovolemic shock. The diagnosis is suspected on the basis of the context of trauma and the clinical examination. Chest X-ray, thoracic ultrasound and CT scan confirm the diagnosis. Chest X-rays identify a volume of blood in excess of 200 to 300 ml.

IV.4.6 Pneumothorax [37]

Pneumothorax is a collection of air in the pleural cavity, occurring in approximately 70% of patients with chest trauma. Tension pneumothorax is a life-threatening condition resulting from the aggravation of a simple pneumothorax. Air is trapped in the pleural cavity, putting pressure on the lung. This leads to compression of the creur and a drop in cardiac output. Chest X-ray and thoracic ultrasound confirm this.

IV.4.7 Pulmonary contusion [38,39].

This alters gas exchange. Patients at high risk of developing acute respiratory distress syndrome (ARDS) can be identified on the basis of the size of the contusion. Unilateral pulmonary contusion rapidly leads to generalized failure of the entire lung. The history of trauma suggests the diagnosis. On the other hand, CT scans systematically reveal it.

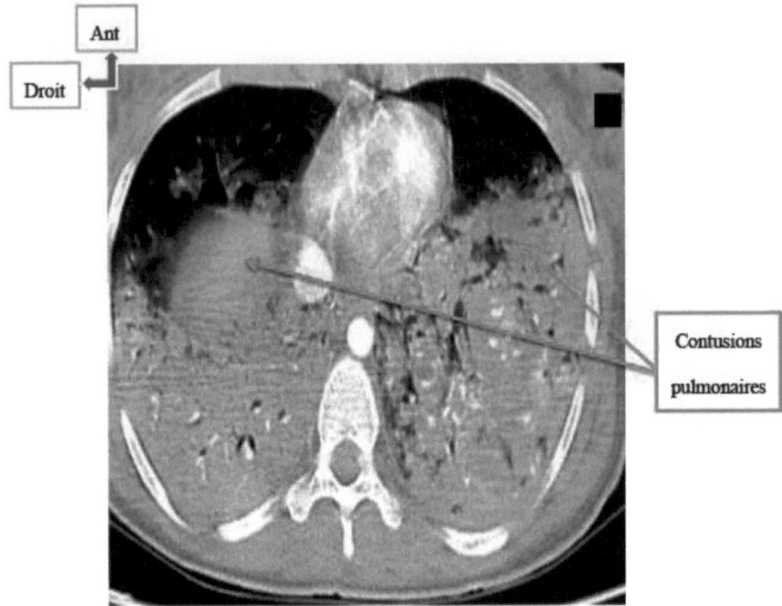

Figure 5: Post-traumatic bilateral pulmonary contusions on CT [25].

IV.4.8 Rupture of the ascending aorta [40-42].

Traumatic rupture of the thoracic aorta is usually caused by direct impact on the sternum. This lesion is also suspected whenever there is a significant transfer of energy. The most common causes of injury are falls of more than 3 metres and accidents occurring at speeds in excess of 50 Km/hr. The clinical examination is normal in around 50% of cases. Chest X-rays are the first step in detection. Computed tomography has a sensitivity of 100% and a specificity of 99.8% for diagnosis.

IV.4.9 Cardiac lesions [42].

The clinical expression of the cardiac lesion remains rare. Contusion of the myocardium is the most common, preferably localized in the right ventricle. Its clinical signs mimic those of cardiac tamponade. Echocardiography is the cornerstone of the diagnostic approach.

IV.4.10 Tracheobronchial lesions [43].

Tracheobronchial lesions are mainly due to penetrating trauma. Over 80% of lesions are located less than 2.5 cm from the carina. There may be subcutaneous emphysema, signs of pneumothorax or pneumomediastinum. In intensive care, a tension pneumothorax generating a continuous air leak despite adequate drainage suggests the diagnosis. Chest X-rays are abnormal in 90% of cases, showing a combination of signs: emphysema, pneumomediastinum, pneumothorax or liquid pleural effusion. CT scans detect more than 90% of tracheal lesions.

IV.4.11 Esophageal lesions [44,45].

The incidence of resophageal lesions varies from 1.2% for firm trauma to 10% for penetrating trauma. The site of the lesion may be cervical (56%), thoracic (30%) or abdominal (17%). Clinical symptoms are rare in intensive care patients. A ruptured resophagus may manifest as Meckler's triad (vomiting, retrosternal pain and subcutaneous emphysema). Chest X-rays are normal in 30% of cases. CT scan shows mediastinal emphysema and fistulas (oeso-pleural or oeso-medianal).

IV.5 Management [20,25,35,46].

The management of thoracic trauma can be dividedëe into two distinct levels of care: prehospital and hospital (in the emergency department and ëventually in the opë^o^ block).

IV.5.1 Pre-hospital management [20]

Data from the initial clinical examination of breathing (respiratory movements and quality^ of breathing) are necessary to recognise major thoracic tesions such as tension pneumothorax, open pneumothorax, costal flap, pulmonary contusion and massive hemothorax. The diagnosis of pneumothorax with marked hëmodynamic instability (hypotension, jugular distension, cyanosis) or suffocating pneumothorax should lead to immëdiate needle dëcompression of the pleural space or exsufflation. And if this does not prove effective on the patient's hëmodynamic state, thoracic drainage must be performed immediately.

IV.5.2 Emergency care [20,25,35,55,49].

IV.5.2.1 Primary balance (ABCDE)

The primary survey using the Advanced Trauma Life Support (ATLS) approach is designed to assess the impact on haematosis, haemodynamics and consciousness, and to implement the first therapeutic measures.

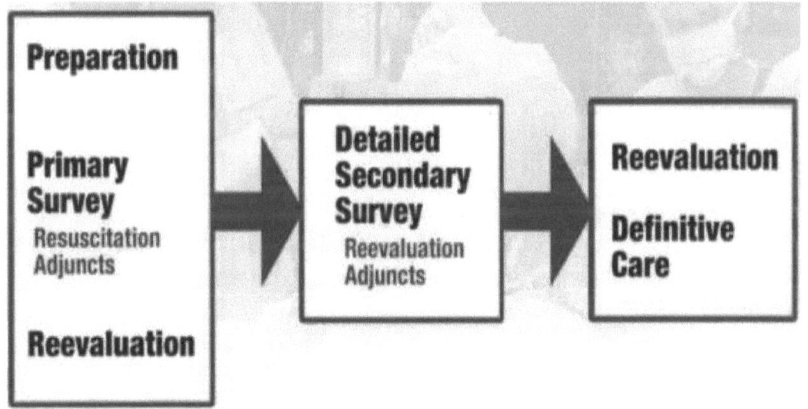

Précautions universelles

Figure 6. Sequence of the primary assessment according to ATLS [55]IV.5.2.1.1 State of the airways

(A)

To assess and ensure the perтëaЫШё of the aërial tract and protection of the cervical spine and prevention of hypoxëmia.

> **Assessment** :

- Search for foreign bodies or trachëe displacement

- Looking for a trauma итуидё.
- Looking for a cervical hëmatoma
- Look for stridor.

> **Gestures** :

- Oxygënothërapie, saturomëtrie
- Aspiration
- Placement of a GUEDEL cannula and nasal trumpet
- Intubation.
- Trachëotomy

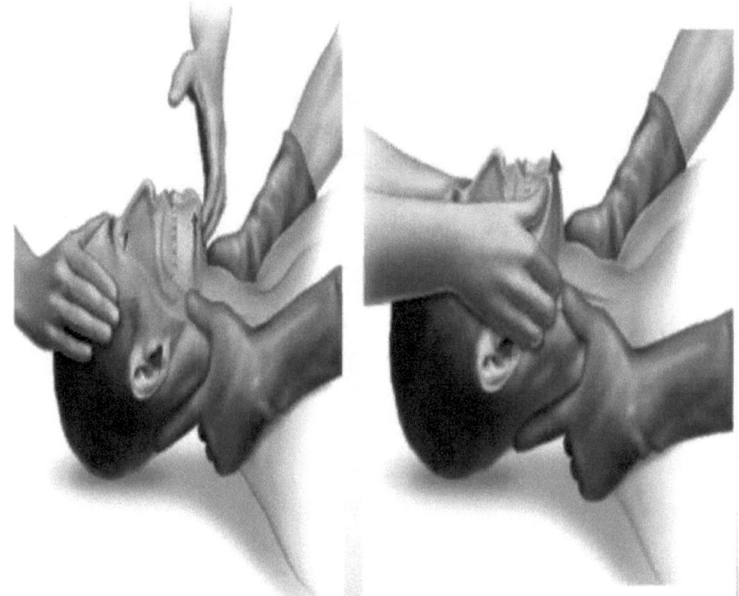

Figure 7. Airway release manoeuvres [55].

IV.5.2.1.2 Respiratory function (B)

Ensure adequate ventilation and oxygenation.

> **Assessment**

- Saturation
- Visual inspection (shortness of breath, cyanosis, intercostal traction, thoraco-abdominal rocking, fluttering of the wings of the nose, sweating) and palpation
- Breathing frequency
- Chest movement
- Auscultation
- Tracheal position

> **Conditions to be identified and addressed during the initial assessment** :

- Pneumotlorax under tension
- Costal flap
- Open pneumotlorax

- Massive hemothorax

IV.5.2.1.3 Traffic (C)

After ruling out tension pneumothorax, any hypotension is hëmorrhagic shock until proven otherwise.

> **Assessment**

- Assess l'ëlal hëmodynamics (blood pressure, pulse, marbling, bleeding syndrome, collapse).
- Assessing awareness
- Skin colouring
- Searching for an exacerbated bleed

> **Gestures** :

- Controlling external hëmorrhage (mechanical hemostasis)
- Two large-calibre venous ports
- Do a cross match, count, lactatemia, gasometry, ionogram
- Rhesus blood grouping
- Vascular filling: 2L of warmed isotonic crystalloi's
- Reassessing the response
- Transfusion if the answer is incorrect.

> **Internal bleeding that may cause shock:**

- Thorax
- Abdomen
- Rëtropëritoine
- Basin
- Fëmur

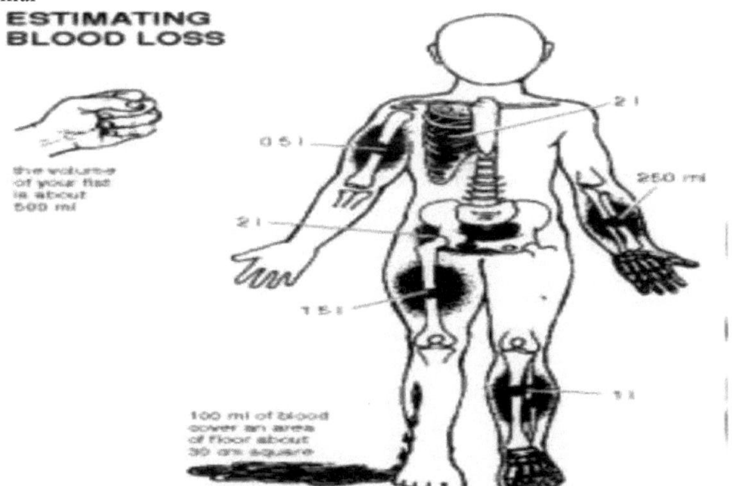

Figure 8. Estimated blood loss by lese territory [Hugh Dudley, Primary Surgery Textbook

]IV.5.2.1.4 State of consciousness (D)

Assess the level of awareness and seek commitment.

> **Assessment and actions**

- Glasgow Decoma Score (GCS)
- Rëponsepupillary
- Defocusing sign
- GCS < 8: intubation
- Change in 1'ëLLI of consciousness: tesion central nervous system but ë rule out intoxication, mëtabolic disorder.

IV.5.2.1.5 Exposure (E)

Look for associated lesions.

> Undress the patient temporarily
> Log Rolling
> Quick summary of lesions
> Prevention of hypothermia

IV.5.2.2 Secondary assessment

The lesion assessment looks for an etiology

> Inspection, where we observe the symmëtria of the thoracic ampliation, look for costal flaps, rib fractures, bruises, wounds, turgidity of the jugular veins.

> Palpation, which reveals subcutaneous cervicothoracic emphysema, pain on movement of the costal grill, movement of a costal flap, peripheral pulses and a decrease in vocal vibrations.

> The percussion by the appreciation of a tympanism or a matite.

> Auscultation reveals asymmetry, abolition of the vesicular murmur, crepitus rales and a focus of alveolar condensation.

The search for associated lesions (skull, spine, thorax, abdomen, pelvis and limbs) is systematic.

IV.5.2.3 Paraclinical examination

IV.5.2.3.1 Biological and functional tests

- The biological work-up will include :
- Haematological work-up: A blood and platelet count to check for deglobulation, a prothrombin level and active partial thromboplastin time to check for disturbances in haemostasis that may be related to bleeding or anticoagulant treatment. Blood grouping and testing for irregular agglutinins with a view to possible transfusion.
- Troponin measurement to detect myocardial contusion
- Arterial gasometry can be used to quantify the level of hypoxia, with a sensitivity of 100% in the diagnosis of severe endothoracic lesions in the context of trauma.
- The Electrocardiogram (ECG) should be performed systëmatically in the patient's bed and if possible during transport. It is a c1ë element of cardiopulmonary monitoring. It can be used to identify right bundle branch block or complete atrioventricular block (compressive pneumothorax), ventricular arrhythmias, signs of myocardial ischaemia (ST-segment elevation) or pulmonary embolism (sinus tachycardia).
- Respiratory function tests (RFTs) are not necessary in an emergency, but after the event to establish the prognosis for respiratory function or diagnose restrictive syndromes.

IV.5.2.3.2 Morphological examinations

The **standard chest X-ray**, with the patient standing and then half-sitting, or at best sitting with deep inspiration and then forced exhalation, is a less sensitive examination, but can detect pleural effusions (greater than 200 cc) and is sufficient to indicate pleural drainage in most cases. If there is a suspicion of polytrauma, a frontal X-ray should be taken with the patient supine and the nasogastric tube in place.
Performing **transparietal ultrasound** in the patient's bed (before mobilisation) in the event of fluid effusion is a rapid procedure, which confirms the diagnosis and repëre with greater certainty the site of insertion. Trans-msophageal echography (TME) demonstrates aortic lesions, pericardial lesions and pneumothorax, among other things, with gene to obtain images. The FAST procedure consists of a shortened thoraco-abdominal ultrasound scan, enabling rapid diagnosis of peritoneal effusion.
Contrast-enhanced **thoracic CT** has many indications in thoracic trauma, but is not recommended in cases of hemodynamic instability. If the patient is well tolerated or clinically stable, a thoracic CT scan with injection is carried out before drainage. This is usually a thoraco-abdomino-pelvic CT scan (TAP-Scan). The indications for CT scans are wide-ranging:

- High-energy firm trauma.
- Mechanism suggestive of serious thoracic lesions (deceleration).
- Serious associated injuries (cranial, abdominal, spinal or pelvic trauma).
- Pre-existing pulmonary pathology.
- Pleural drainage performed without iconography.

IV.5.2.4 Chest drainage

The aim is to re-establish pleural vacuolation in order to remove any intrathoracic organic compression and restore mechanical function to the pleura. The indications for thoracic drainage depend on the nature of the effusion, its volume and its dynamic impact. The indications for thoracic drainage are :

- Suffocating or tension pneumothorax after fine-needle exsufflation
- I leinopneuinothorax indĕpending on their volume and topography
- Occurrence of pneumothorax during mechanical ventilation of any volume
- Complete pneumothorax of the large cavity with pulmonary collapse and/or bilateral and/or symptomatic (painful, respiratory distress, obvious air leak, etc.) regardless of size.
- Hemothorax with a volume greater than 200 mL assessed on CT scan or ultrasound, or the presence on X-ray of a Damoiseau curve or opacity of an entire pulmonary hemichamber after diagnostic pleural puncture.
- Hemothorax with poor respiratory and/or circulatory tolerance.
- Post-traumatic pleural effusion in the presence of pre-existing respiratory pathology leading to poor respiratory tolerance.
- Auto-transfusions in cases of massive hemothorax with major hemodynamic instability if thoracotomy for hemostasis is delayed or not practicable.
- Subcutaneous emphysema without visible pleural detachment in the event of the need for intra- and especially secondary extra-hospital transport where the safety conditions required for quality drainage are not met (asepsis, radiological control, etc.), associated vital lesions which may create diagnostic ambiguity or associated lesions requiring mechanical ventilation and/or general anaesthesia.

The approach to drain insertion may be :

> Anterior: intersection of the second intercostal space (superolateral quadrant of the thorax) and the medio-clavicular line. This is a wide space that avoids the mammary gland and intrathoracic vessels or organs (particularly the internal mammary artery, which runs 2 cm from the edge of the sternum). This insertion site is recommended for pneumothorax.

> Latëral: intersection of the third to fifth intercostal space and the middle or an^terior axillary line, just posterior to the pectoralis major muscle, below this there is a risk of diaphragmatic and/or intra-abdominal tesion. This approach is especially prëconisëe for ëpanchements liquidiens (ëëeHyкë). Some authors may go as far as the 6eme intercostal space.

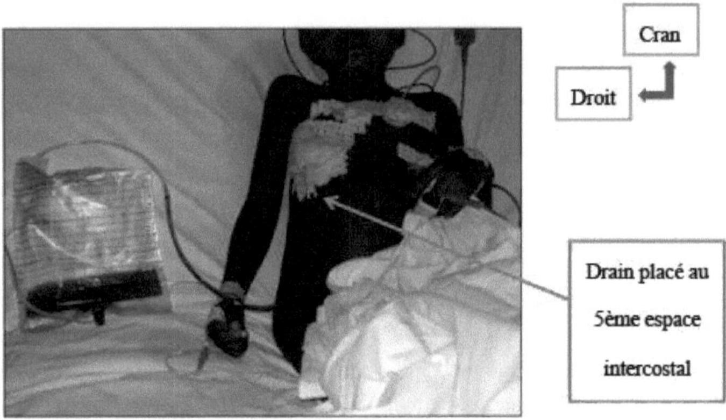

Drain placed in the 5th intercostal space

Figure 9. Chest tube in place at the 5th right intercostal space in a five-year-old child on the second post-operative day of a thoracotomy and decortication [39].

Pleural drains are made of translucent plastic (silicone or plastic) with a diameter of 20 to 40 (5 to 11 mm). The size of the drain depends on the viscosity of the effusion.

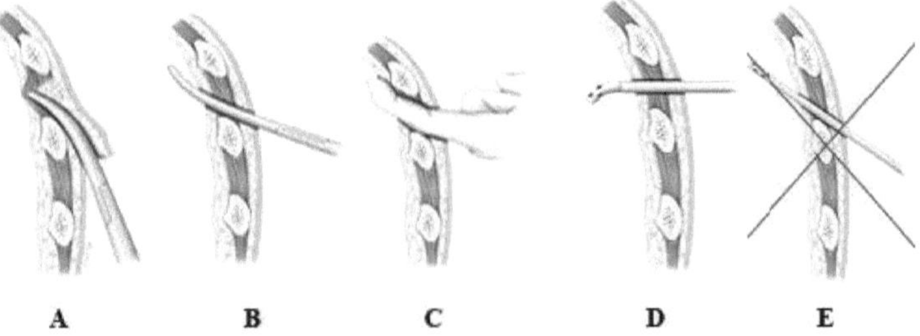

A=Plane-by-plane dissection with Kelly forceps; B=opening of the parietal pleura with Kelly forceps; C=exploring the pleural space with a finger; D=directing the drain into the pleural space using the Monod® insertion cannula; E=No metal trocar chuck.

Figure 14. Technique for placing the pleural drain [35].

A frontal chest X-ray verifies lung re-expansion, the position of the drain and the presence of the most proximal lateral orifice in the pleural space. When inserting the drain in a patient on positive pressure ventilation, some authors suggest disconnecting the patient from the ventilator or, better still, performing an expiratory pause.

IV.5.2.4 General measures

There are two possible situations in an emergency department:

- **Agonic injury :**

Exceptionally, some injured people will be taken to emergency with very severe collapse, respiratory arrest or in a state of apparent death. In the event of success, as evidenced by the restoration of hemodynamics, this procedure is rapidly followed by pleural drainage. Peridural analgesia should always be preferred whenever possible. In the event of signs of haemorrhagic shock, the patient must be transfused or self-transfused (if there is a massive haemothorax) using the residue from the drain collection bag (4 litres in one hour).

- **Temporarily stable injury**

A very systematic approach must be adopted, and the first therapeutic measures must always be implemented, followed by a paraclinical assessment. The patient is given oxygen even in the absence of desaturation, placed in a semi-seated position after a spinal inventory has been carried out, and appropriate analgesia (preferably peridural) is started early, together with external rewarming.

IV.5.2.5 Medical treatment of lesions [2,3].

IV.5.2.2.1 Parietal lesions :

The management of rib fractures is based above all on an appropriate analgesic strategy, in which peridural analgesia plays an important role. In young people, it is essential to look for intrathoracic lesions. Prolonged mechanical ventilation is the first-line treatment for stable costal flaps or those associated with extra-thoracic lesions.

IV.5.2.2.2 Pleuropulmonary lesions :

Hospitalisation is recommended for all patients with pulmonary contusion and its treatment with gënërales measures, fluid restriction and incentive kinesitherapy. A focus of pulmonary contusion, associated with pericontusional edema, is a risk factor for the secondary development of acute respiratory distress syndrome' (ARDS) lesions, especially when associated with hydrosodium overload, massive transfusions, prolonged mechanical ventilation or superinfection. The prevention of post-traumatic pneumonia is achieved by incentive kinesitherapy combined, if necessary, with sequential non-invasive ventilation. There is no benefit to antibiotic prophylaxis in this context. The recognised risk factors for the development of post-traumatic pneumonitis are :

- Age over 50
- Damage to more than five costal arches
- The existence of a costal flap
- The existence of parenchymal contusions visible on the initial X-ray

The treatment for uncomplicated pulmonary hematoma is observation.

IV.5.3 Surgical management [1,2].

IV.5.3.1 Indications for surgical treatment :

According to the recommendations of Advanced Trauma Life Support (ATLS), the indications for thoracotomy are :

> Blood loss from the chest tube collection bag >1,500 ml initially or > 200 ml/hour in 2 to 4 hours or more than 1,500 ml in 24hrs.
> Hemoptysis.
> Massive subcutaneous emphysema.
> Significant air leak through the chest tube.
> Unclear images on chest X-ray or CT scan
> Penetrating chest trauma.

The indications for immediate thoracotomy are :

> Blood loss into the drain collection bag >1,500 ml initially or > 200 ml per hour over 2 to 4 hours.
> Endo-bronchial blood loss, massive pulmonary contusion with significant impairment of mechanical ventilation.
> Lësions of the tracheobronchial tree (major air leak or massive hemothorax).
> Lesion of the creur or large intrathoracic vessels (secondary haemorrhage or pericardial tamponade).

If drainage fails and there is still a clot of more than 500 mL or a third of the hemithorax on X-ray, and at best before 10 days have elapsed, the indication for surgical removal should be discussed.

The indications for rib osteosynthesis are :

> Incarceration of the lung parenchyma or the existence of a bone fragment leading to an intrathoracic organ.
> Major deformations of the wall, especially in young adults, in anticipation of restrictive and painful sequelae.
> Passage osteosynthesis in the case of thoracotomy indicated for intrathoracic organ lesions.
> Primary osteosynthesis of isolated and unstable costal flaps (lateral+++), i.e. not associated with other lesions requiring prolonged sedation, and causing respiratory decompensation despite optimal medical management.

The contraindications to rib osteosynthesis are :

> Association of cranioencephalic trauma with altered consciousness
> Extensive pulmonary contusion complicated by acute respiratory failure
> Spinal and/or medullary lesions

IV.5.3.2 Surgical techniques

> Anterolateral thoracotomy at the level of the 4-6[eme] intercostal spaces is generally recommended. Clamshell (transverse sternotomy and bilateral anterolateral thoracotomy) or semi-Clamshell (longitudinal sternotomy and anterolateral thoracotomy) approaches give better exposure of the thoracic organs.
> The role of minimally invasive surgery in the management of thoracic trauma should neither be underestimated nor overestimated.
> Video-Assisted Thoracospic Surgery or VATS as a pleural space management procëdure in non-critical patients not undergoing massive transfusion can be of great help.

Indications for such an approach include:

- Lësion (penetrating) with little blood loss in a stable patient.

- Persistent haemothorax.
- Empyëme.
- Persistent air leak.
- Suspicion of diaphragmatic rupture

Costal ostëosynthëse is controversial. When it is performed, the most commonly used materials are Judet staples, Borrely slide splints, steel wire, Kirschner wires or screw plates.

IV.5.3.3 Surgical procedures

IV.5.3.3.1 Parietal lesions

Two drains should be inserted during thoracotomy. An antero-superior drain and a postero-inferior drain are classically fixed to the parietal pleural layer, preceded by lavage with warm physiological serum. Costal fractures are rarely indications for osteosynthesis. Only isolated costal flaps giving rise to parietal instability resulting in respiratory failure are eligible for costal osteosynthesis. In other cases, or where there is a contraindication, prolonged mechanical ventilation is the only option. Costal osteosynthesis in the presence of a costal flap is most often a transitional procedure. The thoracotomy must be centred on the flap and wide enough to allow a complete assessment and good exposure of the lesions. The usual approach is a posteroanterior "S" thoracotomy, passing as close as possible to the centre of the flap and, if necessary, enlarged superiorly and posteriorly by means of thoracoplasty with section of the trapezius muscle, known as the Paulson approach.

IV.5.3.3.2 Pleuropulmonary lesions

Tension pneumothorax and open pneumothorax are immediate surgical emergencies. The procedure consists of decompression, endothoracic exploration, treatment of the etiology if possible and placement of drains.

In the event of massive hemotliorax with shock, a hemostasis thoracotomy should be performed. Removal thoracotomy is indicated in the event of persistent hemothorax in excess of 500 cc of blood with clots or a third of the thoracic hemichamber on X-ray, despite well-managed drainage. Delayed hemothorax (formed more than 24 hours after the trauma) often requires a thoracotomy. Video-assisted thoracoscopy (VATS) should be reserved for patients presenting with persistent hemothorax despite well-performed pleural drainage with stable hemodynamics.

Massive pulmonary contusions with significant impairment of mechanical ventilation or ARDS resistant to conservative treatment may be resected to a greater or lesser extent, or circulatory assistance such as extracorporeal membrane oxygenation (ECMO) may be introduced. Simple suturing is the best surgical option for lung lacerations.

IV.5.3.3.3 Tracheobronchial lesions

Tracheal lesions compatible with life are exceptional in thoracic trauma. Bronchial ruptures are less rare. The indication for emergency repair is based on the cardiorespiratory impact, despite thoracic drainage. The standard treatment is suture by thoracotomy.

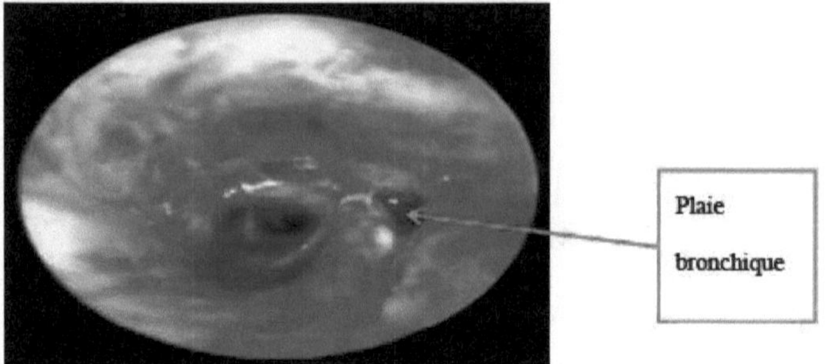

Figure 10. Emergency bronchoscopy showing a bronchial lesion [20].

IV.5.3.3.4 Lesions of the creir and large vessels

Hollow wounds are rare but possible in closed traumatology. They are an absolute surgical emergency. The injured patient must be transferred to the operating theatre as soon as the diagnosis is made. The most frequent clinical presentation is acute aortic insufficiency due to the disinsertion of the aortic valve. Lesions of the large vessels, in particular ruptures of the aortic isthmus, give rise to a clinical picture of sëvëre often fatal hëmorrhagic shock within 30 minutes, which is generally a very short time for any surgical procedure.

IV.5.3.3.5 Lesions of the resophagus

A per-endoscopic surgical procedure is possible, especially in the case of a resophageal foreign body, but in the vast majority of cases a thoracotomy or even a laparotomy is required. In cases of deep laceration or perforation of the upper resophagus (cervical or thoracic), the reference approach is a posterior thoracotomy followed by suture (laceration) or resection and anastomosis (perforation). For lesions of the lower resophagus (abdominal), an anterior thoracotomy coupled with a transverse xiphoid incision or even a supra-umbilical laparotomy is recommended. However, in the event of peritonitis due to resophageal perforation, a xiphopubic laparotomy should be performed in conjunction with the thoracotomy.

IV.5.3.3.6 Diaphragmatic ruptures and hernias

An emergency exploratory and curative laparotomy should be performed as soon as possible. The xypho-pubic incision is preferred. The large peritoneal cavity is washed with warmed saline and the diaphragm sutured. An associated median sternotomy is sometimes necessary. In cases of diaphragmatic hernia, the approach is either abdominal or thoracic. The procedure involves reduction of the hernia contents, resection and closure of the sac, with or without the use of a prosthesis.

IV.6 Evolution and prognosis [25,47].

The main complications associated with thoracic trauma are respiratory failure, pneumonia, respiratory distress and pachypleuritis. They are directly correlated with the severity of the trauma and the patient's comorbidities.

Hemothoraxes can become clots, which at best will result in pachypleuritis with fibrothorax and at worst purulent pleurisy. Finally, at a later stage, diaphragmatic eventrations may be responsible (most often on the left) for strangulation of the digestive contents herniated through the diaphragm and perforation of a hollow organ in the thorax recognised beforehand.

Pneumothorax with significant air leakage (large pulmonary wound or direct tracheobronchial involvement) can result in the heart pump being damaged and the injured person dying.

In the short term, pneumonia is the most common complication of pulmonary contusion. In the long term, survivors of multiple trauma with thoracic trauma have functional limitation as evidenced by 70% of patients with altered respiratory function tests.

The vital prognosis is predicted by polytrauma severity scores. The most widely used is the Injury Severity Score or its аЬrёдё l'Abbreviate Injury Score (AIS). The AIS determines the short-, medium- and long-term prognosis, as well as the need for ventilation and its duration. It is used to classify trauma patients into two groups:

- I- **1<ISS<16:** LCger a modCrC
- **16 < ISS < 25 :** SCrieux
- **1-25 < ISS < 50 :** SCvere
- I- **50 < ISS < 75 :** Critical
- I- **75**= Maximum

The AIS ëva1ue the local sëvëritë of the trauma. A thoracic AIS score greater than or equal to 4 defines the thoracic injury as being at least severe or even maximal (if greater than 6). ARDS, a serious complication and the leading cause of death following thoracic trauma, has been the subject of an American-European consensus. It is a predictive score for the occurrence and prognosis of ARDS. It is called the Thoracic Trauma Severity Score (TTSS) and ranges from 0 to 25.

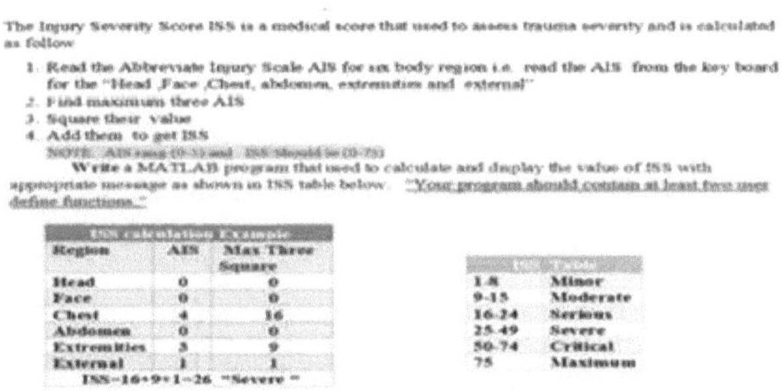

The Injury Severity Score ISS is a medical score that used to assess trauma severity and is calculated as follow

1. Read the Abbreviate Injury Scale AIS for six body region i.e. read the AIS from the key board for the "Head ,Face ,Chest, abdomen, extremities and external"
2. Find maximum three AIS
3. Square their value
4. Add them to get ISS

Write a MATLAB program that used to calculate and display the value of ISS with appropriate message as shown in ISS table below. "Your program should contain at least two user define functions."

Region	AIS	Max Three Square
Head	0	0
Face	0	0
Chest	4	16
Abdomen	0	0
Extremities	3	9
External	1	1
ISS=16+9+1=26 "Severe"		

1-8	Minor
9-15	Moderate
16-24	Serious
25-49	Severe
50-74	Critical
75	Maximum

Figure 11. AIS and ISS scores [48]

Table I: Revised Trauma Score (RTS) [51].

RTS (Revised trauma scored					
Signs	0	1	2	3	4
Consciousness (Glasgow coma scale)	3	4-5	6-8	9-12	13-15
Systolic blood pressure	0	1-49	50-75	76-89	>89
Respiration rate	0	1-5	6-9	>29	10-29

RTS = 0.9368 (GCS) + 0.7326 (BPs) + 0.2908 (RR)

Minimal score = 0, corresponds to the survival rate = 2,7%.

Maximal score = 7,8408, corresponds to the survival rate = 99%.

The injured patients with the score less than 4 might be transported immediately with the red marking.

8. Publications on the subject

8.1 In the world

In 1989, in the United States, *Lociero et al* [51], after a retrospective study over five years, found that traffic accidents (48%) followed by suicide (29%) and homicide (22%) were the main causes of trauma. The overall mortality rate was 18%, of which 20% was attributable to thoracic trauma. The main mechanism of injury was acceleration-deceleration phenomena. The thoracic lesions observed were: rib fractures (45%), flail chest (5%), pneumothorax (25%), hemothorax (25%), pulmonary lesions (26%). Trauma to the limbs (46%) was the most common associated injury. 150 patients (15%) underwent thoracotomy.

In 2000, in the United States of America, *Kulshrestha et al* [13] found that 98% of thoracic injuries were firm. They found that fractures of the first and second ribs (49%), pneumothorax (20%), pulmonary contusion (12%) and lesion of a thoracic vessel (6%) were the major thoracic lesions. Approximately 18% of patients benefited from thoracic drainage and just under 7% from thoracotomy.

In 2001, in Belgium, *Segers et al* [52], following a retrospective study of 187 patients, found a sex ratio of 2.9M:1F and an average age of 41.1 years. Road traffic accidents (72.2%) and falls (17.1%) were the main causes of thoracic trauma. The mean Injury Severity Score was 27.5 ±7. Thoracic trauma was isolated in 17.6% of cases. Rib fractures (n=133; 71.1%), pulmonary contusion (n=110; 58.8%) and pneumothorax (n=78; 41.17%) were the main thoracic injuries. They found that 19 patients (10.2%) benefited from thoracic drainage and 11 patients (5%) from thoracotomy. Conservative treatment alone (61%) was the main management modality. Pneumonia (38%) and acute respiratory distress syndrome (7%) were the two most common complications. The mortality rate was 16.6%.

8.2 In Africa

In 2016, in Ethiopia, *Getachew et al* [53], following a descriptive cross-sectional study

In a retrospective study, the prevalence of thoracic trauma in Addis Ababa was 9.5%. The sex ratio was 3H/1F and the mean age was 28 ±10 years. Pedestrians (69%) were the main victims. Trauma to the limbs (51%) and head trauma (20%) were the two main associated injuries.

In 2018, in Nigeria, *Okonta et al* [54], in a four-year prospective study of 126 patients, found 104 men (82.5%) and 22 women (17.54%) with a sex ratio of 4.7:1. The mean age was 40.4 ±10 years. Subcutaneous emphysema (n=39; 31%), rib fractures (n=69; 54.8%), pulmonary contusion (n=73; 57.9%), hemothorax (n=26; 20.6%) and pneumothorax (n=16; 12.7%) were the main thoracic lesions. Trauma to the limbs (n=25; 19.8%), cranio-medullary trauma (n=17; 13.5%) and abdominal trauma (n=13; 10.3%) were the most common associated lesions. Conservative treatment alone was used in 36.5% of cases and 63.5% of patients benefited from thoracic drainage. The main complication was respiratory distress syndrome (8.7%).

8.3 In Cameroon

From 1er January 1991 to 31 December 2003 at the Yaounde Central Hospital (HCY), *Chichom et al* [19] conducted a retrospective study of 354 patients. Of these, 286 were men and 68 women, with a sex ratio of 4.2:1. The mean age was 41.9±16.3 years. Traffic accidents (63.6%) were the most frequent cause of thoracic trauma. The main thoracic lesions were rib fractures (n=178 ;50.5%), hëmothorax (n=137 ;38.7%) and pneumothorax (n=48 ;13.5%). Trauma to the limbs (n=119 ;33.6%) and neurotrauma (n=87 ;24.6%) represented the first two associated lesions. Management modalities ëwere respectively conservative treatment alone in 164 patients (46.3%), thoracic drainage employed in 164 patients (46.3%) and thoracotomy performed in 51 patients (14.4%). The overall mortality rate was 7.6%.

At the CHUY, *ZOA et al* [55], in their final dissertation, noted that of the 31 patients studied, the sex ratio was four men to one woman. The mean age was 31.92±12.74. Students (18.92%) were the most common occupation. The hospital frequency of thoracic trauma was 7.85% in 2016 and 7.53% in 2017. The circumstances of occurrence were dominated by road accidents (48.65%). Pulmonary contusions (48.65%) were the most frequent lesions and polytrauma was found in 6 patients (12%). Conservative treatment combined with thoracic drainage (91.9%) was the main management modality. Thoracotomy was performed in 16.2% of cases. No deaths were recorded.

V- METHODOLOGY

V.1 Type of study

We тепё a descriptive cross-sectional study with retrospective data collection.

V.2 Study locations

V.2.1 Description of the Yaounde Emergency Centre (CURY)

This is a second-category hospital created in 2015. It is located in the MESSA district in the 2nd arrondissement of Yaounde. It shares borders with Yaounde's central hospital and is opposite the latter, the headquarters of the Expanded Programme on Immunisation (EPI). The centre specialises in managing emergencies and transferring patients to other hospitals for further treatment. It has a capacity of fifty beds, which can be extended to one hundred. It employs around two hundred and fifty-six people, including general practitioners, nurses, various specialists (a thoracic surgeon, visceral surgeons, neurosurgeons, internists, anaesthetists, etc.), paramedical and administrative staff. It is made up of a number of different units, including the trauma and non-trauma units, the primary care area, hospital wards, the intensive care unit, the archives and other sub-units.

V.2.2 Description of Yaounde University Hospital (CHUY)

The Centre Hospitalier Universitaire de Yaounde is located in the city of Yaounde, in a district of the 6th arrondissement called MELEN at a place called TOTAL MELEN. It is a first class university hospital. It covers all the main medical specialities. The emergency department is the gateway for all patients to the CHUY. It is a medical-surgical department and includes a scrub room and minor surgery. The department has a capacity of 4 beds, two observation rooms, the first of which has 3 beds (not currently operational) and the second has 8 beds. It is one of the main hospitals where medical students do their clinical training. The hospital's surgical unit comprises five wards: two inpatient wards, a nurses' ward, an office for the head nurse and an office for the residents in each ward.

V.3. Duration and period of the study

Our study covered a period of 7 months, from 1 January 2021 to 30 June 2021. Our study period was from 1er January 2016 to 31 December 2020.

V.4. Study population

V .4.1-source population

It consisted of all trauma patient files of all types from 1 January 2016 to 31 December 2020 at CURY and CHUY.

V .4.2-Target population

It was made up of all the records of patients presenting with at least one post-traumatic thoracic lesion suspected clinically or detected on thoracic imaging during the study period.

V .4.3- Inclusion criteria

Have ttt included in our study,

❖ Records of patients hospitalized for a clinically suspected post-traumatic thoracic lesion or discovered after thoracic imaging of the 1's of entry or during their hospitalization during the study period.

V.4.4-Non-inclusion criteria

- Patients whose records did not include information on age, sex, cause of trauma, mechanism of injury, nature of thoracic injury or treatment modalities.
- Records of patients discharged against medical advice

V.5-Sampling

V.5.1 Sampling method

Our sample was random and not exhaustive.

V.5.2 Minimum sample size

The formula we used to calculate the minimum sample size was the **Cochrane** formula [55] :

$$n = \frac{\left(Z1-\frac{\alpha}{2}\right)^2 x\, p\, x\,(1-p)}{e^2}$$

n = minimum sample size

Z 1-a/2 = abscissa of the normal distribution curve whose value of the area under the curve corresponds to the confidence level dtsirt. For a confidence level of 95% and a margin of error of 5% such as йхёе conventionally in santë research, this value is 1.96.

P = prevalence of Гёуёпетеп!: ётudiё in the population that is 1^studied.

According to Getachew et al. in Ethiopia in 2016, thoracic injuries accounted for 9.5% of all injuries [53].

Numëric application:

$$N = \frac{(1{,}96)^2 x\, 0{,}095\, x\,(1-0{,}095)}{0{,}05^2}$$

N=330.028156 or approximately 330.

We then obtained a minimum sample size of 330 patient records.

V.6. Study variables

> **Socio-demographic data:** age, gender, occupation, insurance policy.

> **Clinical data :** Place of incident, existence of a notion of rëfërence, dëtime before hospital arrest, cause of trauma, tesional mëcanism, type of trauma, comorbid^, primary workup (ёlяl of the aërial tracts, arërial pressure, respiratory rate, cardiac rate, Glasgow coma score, oxygëne saturation), nature of thoracic tesion and associated tesions, site with the most ёкуё AIS score, thoracic AIS score, ISS score.

> **Paraclinical data:** Chest X-ray and report, thoracic CT scan and report, thoracic ultrasound (mode and report), bronchoscopy and report, other functional/morphological investigations and report, lK'moglobin level, creatinine level.

> **Therapeutic information :** Resuscitation measures (vascular filling, ventilation, oxygënothërapy, external cardiac massage, vasopressive drugs, cardiotonics, blood transfusion), respiratory kiiK'sithK'rapy, transfusion, analgesia (type, level, route of administration), antibiotic prophylaxis and antibiotics used, corticosteroid therapy, gastric protection, types of surgery (thoracotomy, parietal suture, other), indication for thoracotomy, thoracic drainage (type, insertion site, time to removal), exsufflation.

> **Prognostic data:** length of hospital stay, complications after conservative treatment

(pneumonia, ARDS), post-opëratatory complications (secondary bleeding, parietal sepsis, empyema, reinterventions, cardiac arrest), vital prognosis (survival or dëcës).

> **Assessment of the association between variables and specific treatment modalities:** A $p<0.05$ ë1эк value is considered to be a statistically significant association and in these cases the Odd Ratios (ORs) have ë1ë dëterminës.

The frequency of emergency admissions for thoracic trauma per year has ë1ë been calculated according to the following formula:

Number of patients with at least one post-traumatic lesion of the thorax over one year Total number of patients admitted to emergency departments for all types of trauma over one year

n = - N

V.7. Equipment

The material required for our study included the following for the collection and analysis of the data collected:

V.7.1. Recording equipment

- A data sheet to be completed by the investigator. It will contain data on patient age, sex, tesional mechanism, primary work-up, tesional work-up, results of morphological examinations carried out, management methods, patient progression and length of hospitalisation.
- Two registers: one for each hospital
- A scientific calculator
- Three blue and red ballpoint pens
- Four 2B pencils
- An eraser
- A ream of A4 paper
- A laptop computer and tëlëphone

V.7.2 Data analysis equipment

- Microsoft Word and Excel
- Statistical tools (SPSS version 23.0, CS Pro 7.6.0 and MS Excel 2019)

V.8. Data collection procedure and statistical analysis

We collected and analysed the data according to the following ëstages:

- **Step 1:** Throughout February 2021, we visited the emergency department of the Yaounde University Hospital. During the first week, we sorted the files of trauma patients with at least one thoracic lesion in the period from 1er January 2016 to 31 December 2020. During the other three weeks, we recorded the data collected on our data sheet.
- **Step 2:** During the months of March, April and May 2021, we went to the emergency department of the Yaounde Emergency Centre. During the first week, we sorted the records of trauma patients with at least one thoracic lesion in the period from 1 January 2016 to 31 December 2020. During the following weeks, we recorded the data collected on our data sheet.
- **Stage 3:** From 01 June to 21 June 2021, we analysed the data using SPSS 23.0 software from the database created using CsPro 7.6 software. Firstly, the analysis was

univariate (numbers and frequencies). It was then bivariate (p-value and OR calculations). Finally, binary logistic regression was used to search for independent associated factors (adjusted p-value and adjusted OR calculations).

❖ **Stage 4:** From 21 June to 10 July 2021, we compiled the results in the form of tables and graphs in MS Word and MS Excel 2019.

V.9. Dissemination of results

The results and conclusions of our study will be disseminated to the general public via social media and the written press.

V.10. Definition of operational terms

❖ **Thoracic trauma:** injury to the chest wall or an intrathoracic organ [1].

❖ **Polytrauma**: the presence of at least two physical lesions or organ systems, one of which may be life-threatening, leading to physical, cognitive or psychosocial dysfunction and functional disability [2].

❖ **Penetrating trauma to the thorax:** open Lësion limited superiorly by the neck and inferiorly by the lower costal margin with effraction of the parietal plevre [25].

❖ **Firm trauma to the thorax:** Lësion of the chest wall or an intrathoracic organ without invasion of the pariëtal plevre [25].

❖ **Hemothorax:** effusion of blood into the pleural space [25].

❖ **Pneumothorax**: aëric effusion into the pleural space [25].

❖ **Thoracic drainage :** Evacuation of pleural fluid abnormal in nature, volume and/or appearance by means of a drain ркcë in 1 pleural space [25].

❖ **Odd Ratio (OR):** Ratio of the odds of a ëvënement occurring to a group A of individuals, for example a disease, to that of the same ëvënement occurring to a group B of individuals [47].

❖ **Acute respiratory distress syndrome (ARDS):** Inflammatory process affecting the airways leading to lesional pulmonary edema characteriscdërisë by chronic respiratory failure lasting less than a week, bilateral alveolar-interstitial opacities visible on chest imaging, profound hypoxemia (PaO2/FiO2 ratio less than or equal to 300 mmHg) and absent or minimal hydrostatic involvement [49].

❖ **Simple thoracic contusion:** Existence of a notion of shock to the chest wall with low energy transfer (reduced speed trauma, no shock wave), chest pain of intensity^ ЫДёге a modërëe without tachyp^e or other tesion on clinical examination [57].

V .9. Ethical considerations

We obtained ethical clearance after submission of this work to the Com^ d'Ethique Institutionnel de la recherche pour de la santë humaine de l'universte de Douala (CEI-UDo). Then, following requests, the heads of the two study hospitals granted us research authorisations. And, in compliance with the Nuremberg code (1996) and the dëc1aration of Helsinki (2013), our ëtude was conducted with strict respect for dignity without interfering with patient follow-up.

VI - RESULTS

From ı January 2016 to 31 December 2020, **17275** patients ële reguired at CURY and CHUY combiires emergency departments, including **11761** for trauma indëpendent of location.

These include:

> **1785** had at least one post-traumatic thoracic lesion.

> **965** patients had medical records with missing data

usable anamnestic or management data

> **462** patients had left hospital against medical advice.

> **358** patients, who met all our inclusion criteria and for whom we were able to

The files entered in our study were ë1.ë.

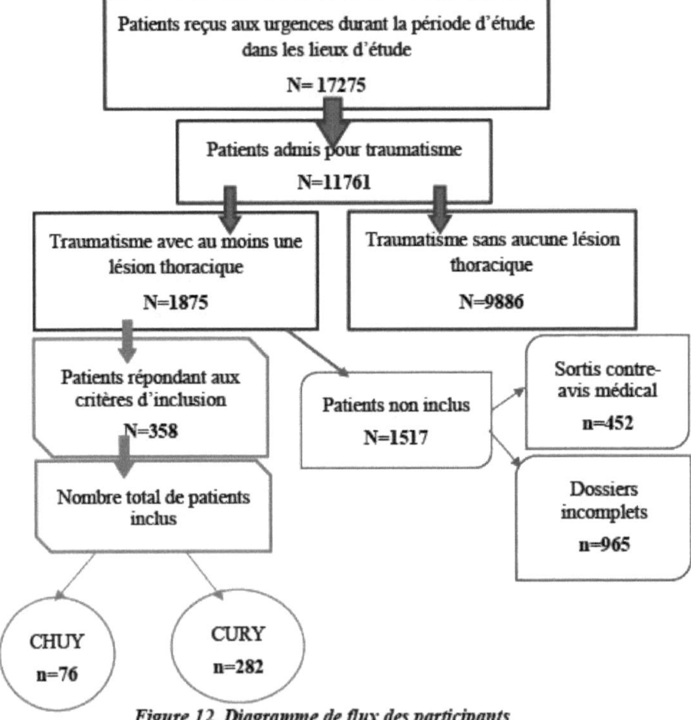

Figure 12. Diagramme de flux des participants

Figure 12. Participant flow diagram

VI.1 Epidemiological profile of our study population

VI.1.1 Socio-demographic characteristics

We had coШдё 358 patient records of which 296 ëwere men and 62 were women i.e. a sex ratio of 5H/1F.

The mëdian age ëик of 30 [23-40] years and extremes of 1 and 96 years.

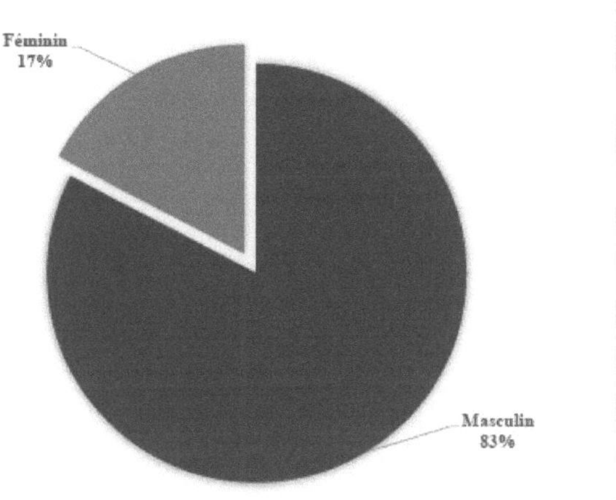

Figure 13. Breakdown of patients by gender

The 20-40 age group (n=215; 60.1%) was the most represented (Figure 19).

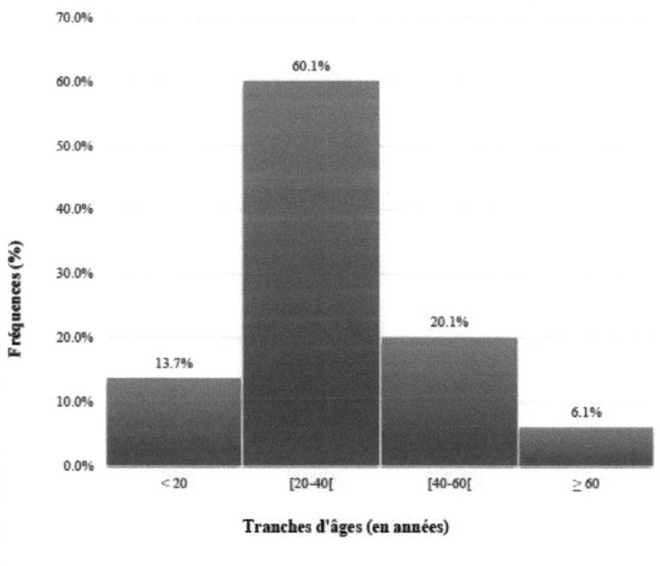

Figure 14. Breakdown of patients by age group (in years)

The informal sector (58.4%) was the most common occupational sector.
Most patients were uninsured (see Table II).

Table II: Breakdown by occupation and insurance policy

Variables	Numbers (N=358)	Percentages (%)
Profession		
Informal sector	209	**58,4**
Student	43	12,0
Private sector	37	10,3
Civil servant	27	7,5
Student	17	4,8
Retirement	15	4,2
No profession	10	2,8
Insurance policy	23	**6,4**

VI.1.2 Frequency per year of thoracic trauma in emergency departments in the study sites.

We have used the following formula to carry out the calculations

Number of patients with at least one post-traumatic lesion of the thorax in one year n Total number of patients admitted to emergency departments for all types of trauma in one year N

The average overall frequency of chest injuries was 16.5%, with a peak in 2019 (24.4%). The frequency of thoracic trauma was higher at CURY than at CHUY in all study years except 2016, as shown in the figure above.

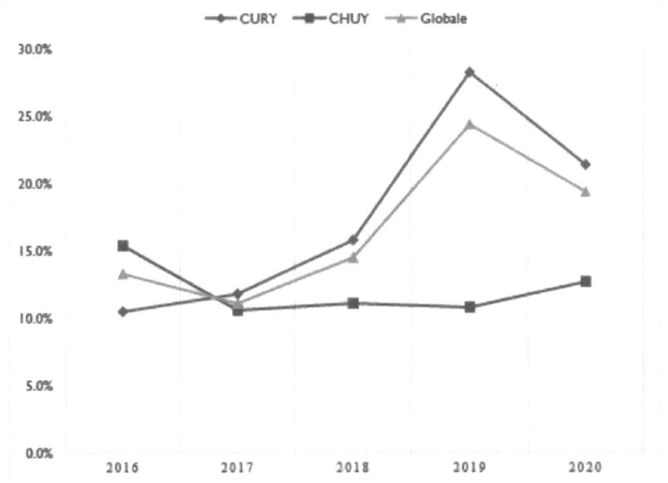

Figure 15. Frequency of thoracic trauma by year from 2016 to 2020 (N=358)

VI.2 Clinical and paraclinical profiles of victims

VI.2.1. Clinical characteristics

The vast majority of incidents took place in Yaoundë (91.0%). Unmedicalised transport (93.6%) was the most frequent.

Arterial hypertension (55.7%) was the most common comorbidity.

Table III: Breakdown of casualties according to the context of the transport and the comorbidities

Variables	Numbers (N=358)	Percentages (%)
Incident location		
Yaounde	326	**91.0**
Less than 100 km from Yaounde	16	4.5
100Km or more from Yaounde	16	4.5
Number of patients referred	64	**17,9**
Means of transport		
Non-medical	335	**93,6**
Medicalise	23	6,4
Comorbidities	88	**24,5**
Arterial hypertension	49	**55,7**
Alcoholism over 40g a day	23	26,1
Diabetes	12	13,6
Smoking	10	8,8
Epigastralgia	4	4,5
IRC[1]	1	1,1
HIV[2]	1	1,1
Pregnancy	1	1,1

Victims more frequently (59.5%) went to the emergency department less than 3 hours after the trauma occurred.

The mëdian time between the moment of trauma and arrival at the emergency ëlaк **of 2[1-4] hours** and extremes of **1** and **800 hours**.

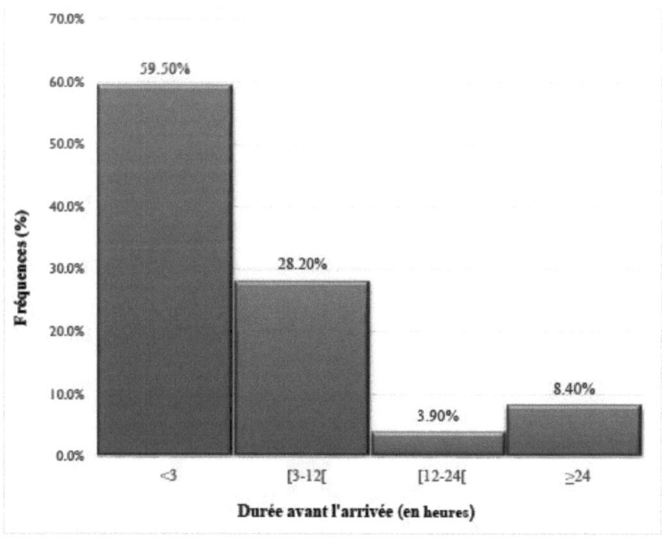

[1]=Chronic Respiratory Failure

[2]=Human Immunodeficiency Virus

Figure 16. Breakdown of patients by length of time to arrival at A&E (N=358)

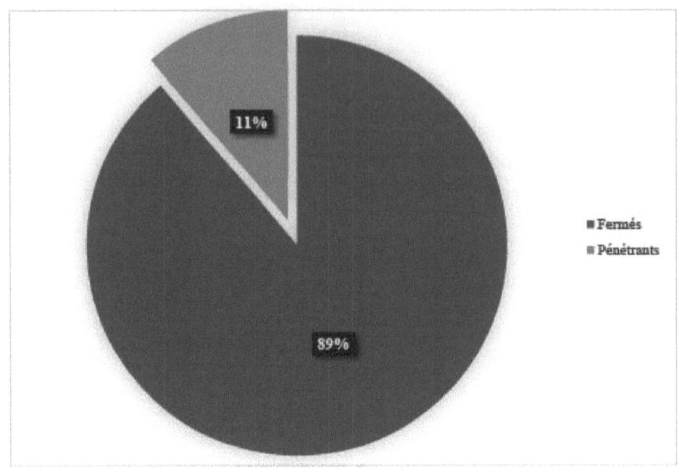

Figure 17. Distribution of patients by type of trauma (N=358)

Most thoracic injuries were firm (89%).

Traffic accidents (60.3%) were the most frequent cause.

Motorbike accidents (62.0%) were the most frequent.

Table IV: Breakdown of patients according to circumstances of onset

Variables	Number (N=358)	Percentage (%)
Causes of trauma		
Traffic accident	216	**60,3**
Aggression/rights	61	**17,0**
Domestic accident	51	**14,2**
Accident at work	20	5,6
Suicide attempt	7	2,0
Other	3	0,9
Type of traffic accident (n=216)		
Vëhicle-vëhicle	130	**60,3**
Vëvehicle only	48	22,0
Vëhicle-piëton	38	17,7
Type of vehicle damaged (n=216)		
Motorbike	134	**62,0**
Automotive	59	27,3
Truck	15	7,0
Bus	8	3,7
Patient position in case of vehicle-vehicle (n=130)		
Passenger	72	**55,4**

Driver	58	44,6

*Others=Sports accident and mob justice

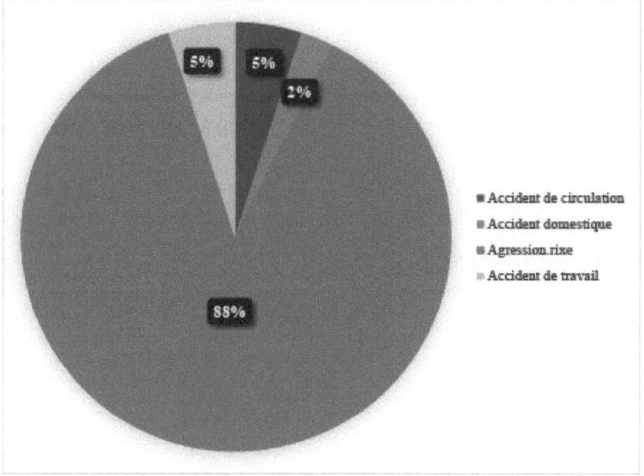

Figure 18. Breakdown of causes of penetrating trauma (n=40)

Stabbings were the main cause of head injuries (cf.
Figure 22).
Dĕcĕlĕration (48.3%) ĕlɯl: the most frequent tesional mĕcaɯsm.
The dagger (86.3%) ĕlɯl: 1 stabbing weapon most frequently тсптгёе.

Tableau V: Breakdown of casualties by injury mechanism

Variables	Numbers (N=358)	Percentages (%)
Lesion mechanisms		
Dĕcĕlĕration	173	**48,3**
White weapon	51	14,2
Compression	46	12,8
Drop	33	9,2
Ingestion of caustic	19	5,3
Hits	13	3,6
Inhalation of a foreign body	9	2,6
Firearm	5	1,4
Other	9	2,6
Type of knife (n=51)		
Dagger	44	**86,3**
Bottle shards	4	7,8
Machete	2	3,9
Glass shards	1	2,0
Nature of foreign body (n=9)		
Carbon monoxide	5	**55,6**

Feed	3	33,3
Object	1	11,1

*Others=Burn, ëlectrification, lacëration, ëtirement.

Most patients had unobstructed aërial tracts (92%).

Shock was observed in 10.3% of patients.

Tableau VI: Characteristics of primary balance parameters

Variables	Numbers (N=358)	Percentages (%)
Airways		
Free	329	**91,9**
Obstructed	29	8,1
Respiratory rate (cycles/minute)		
<12	5	1,4
[12-21[	64	17,9
[21-30[	179	50,0
>30	110	30,7
Heart rate (beats/minute)		
<60	8	2,2
[60-100[	142	39,7
[100-120[	141	39,4
>120	67	18,7
Systolic blood pressure (mmHg)		
<90	38	**10,6**
[90-130[	144	40,2
[130-140[	73	20,4
>140	103	28,8
Glasgow score		
3 a 8	17	4,7
9 a 12	18	5,1
13 a 15	323	**90,2**
Oxygen saturation (%)		
<80	22	6,1
[80-90[	23	6,4
[90-96[	93	26,0
>96	220	61,5

The mëdian Revised Trauma Score (RTS) **was 7.84** with an interquartile range [7.557.84] and extremes ranging **from 1.96** to **7.84**.

Tableau VII: Breakdown of the primary balance as a function of central tendency parameters

Variables	Average (±ET)	Median (IIQ)	Min-Max
Breathing rate (in cycles/minute)	-	26,0 (22,0-31,5)	4-88
Heart rate (beats/minute)	-	102,0 (89,0-114,0)	32-191

Systolic blood pressure (mmHg)	-	129,0 (114,0-141,0)	40-206
Glasgow Coma Score	-	15,0 (15,0-15,0)	3-15
Oxygen saturation (%)	-	96,0 (94,0-98,0)	33-99
Revised Trauma Score (RTS)	-	7,84 (7,55-7,84)	1,96-7,84

Thoracic ksions ëtended to be single (70.1%).

Pulmonary contusion (65.3%) ë-was the most common thoracic ksion.

Table VIII: Characteristics of thoracic lesions

Variables	Numbers (N=358)	Percentages (%)
Number of thoracic lesion(s)		
Unique	251	**70,1**
Multiple	107	29,9
Nature of the lesion		
Pulmonary contusion	234	**65,3**
Rib fractures	95	36,8
Simple thoracic contusion	83	23,2
I kmothorax	68	19,0
Pneumothorax	41	11,5
Non-pënëtrating wound	37	10,3
Costal flap	31	8,7
Emphysëme sub-cuta^	18	5,0
ffisophagitis	17	4,7
Lësion of the heart*	13	3,6
TraclK'o-bronchial lësion	10	3,58
A^olary kmorrhage	7	2,0
Sternal fracture	6	1,7
Burn of the airways**	6	1,7
Diaphragmatic rupture	1	0,3
Rupture of the aorta	1	0,3
Other	4	1,4

*Lësions cardiaques= Myocardial contusion, rhythm disorders, conduction disorders, përicardial tamponade, myocardial infarction, valvulopathy.

**Bru l ure des voies aëriennes=inha l ation d'un corps etranger entrainant une perte de substance de la muqueuse des voies aëriennes hautes et basses.

***Others=cutaneous bruising, pinching of an intercostal nerve and parietal abscess.

Haemothorax (80%) was the most frequent lesion after penetrating trauma (C.f figure 23).

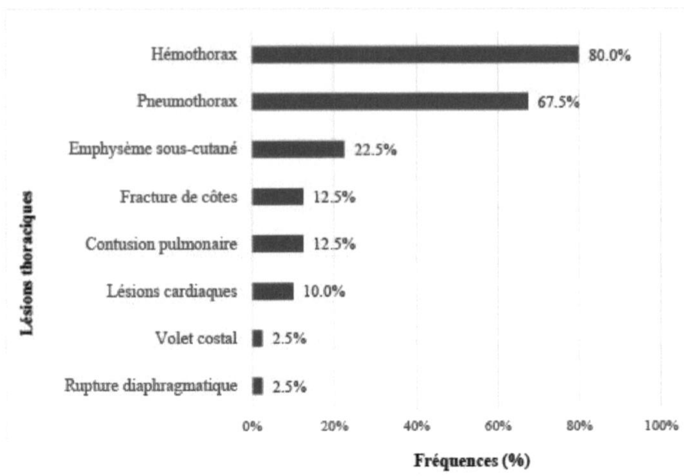

Figure 19. Distribution of thoracic injuries secondary to penetrating trauma (n=40)

Cranioencephalic trauma (56.6%) was the most common associated lesion. The Injurity Severity Score (ISS) mëdian ëla11 of **20 [13-41]** and extremes ranging from **4** to **75.** The majority of patients (32.5%) had severe ISS.

Table IX: Characteristics of associated lesions and Injury Severity Score

Variables	Numbers (N=358)	Percentages (%)
Presence of an associated lesion	**265**	**74,0**
Number of associated lesions (n=265)		
A lesion	156	**58,9**
Two lesions	76	28,7
More than two lesions	33	12,4
Location of associated lesions (n=265)		
Cranioencephalic	**150**	**56,6**
Lower limb	58	21,9
Abdomen	48	18,1
Senior member	55	15,4
Face	35	13,2
Basin	32	12,1
Spine	29	10,9
Neck	9	3,4
Injury Severity Score (n=265)		
<16*	73	27,5
16 a 24**	67	25,3
25 a 49***	86	32,5
50 a 74****	31	11,7
75*****	8	3,0

*=Leger to moderate

**=Serieux
***=Severe
****=Criticism
*****=Maximal

VI.2.2. Paraclinical characteristics

The standard chest X-ray (90.5%) was the most common morphological examination.

Table X: Characteristics of paraclinical examinations

Variables	Numbers (N=358)	Percentages (%)
Chest X-ray	324	**90,5**
Blood count and formula	305	85,2
Measuring creatinemia	113	31,2
Chest scan	76	21,2
Pleural ultrasound	45	12,6
Echo mode FAST (n=45)	40	88,9
Upper gastrointestinal endoscopy	10	1,1
Electrocardiogram	13	19,5
Echocardiography	7	3,58
Bronchial endoscopy	4	3,6

VI.3 Methods of therapeutic management of thoracic trauma and their results

Medical treatment alone **(69.9%)** was the most common treatment modality.
Thoracotomy was performed on **7.3%** of victims (see Table XII).

Table XI: Breakdown of patients according to specific lesion management methods

Variables	Numbers (N=358)	Percentages (%)
Terms and conditions		
Medical treatment alone	250	**69,9**
Medical treatment combined with drainage pleural	46	12,8
Thoracotomy	26	**7,3**
Other types of surgery	36	10,0

***Others** = suturing and trimming of wounds, per-endoscopic procedures (removal of foreign bodies), drainage of abscesses, laparotomy (diaphragmatic rupture).

Persistent lethargy (42.3%) was the most frequent indication for thoracotomy.
The postëro-latëral route (50.0%) was the most common approach.
Lung resection (69.2%) was the most frequent surgical procedure (see Table XIII).

Table XII: Thoracotomy characteristics

Variables	Number (n=26)	Percentages (%)
Indications for thoracotomy		
Persistent haemothorax	11	**42,3**
Unstable costal flap	9	34,6
Massive pulmonary contusion	3	11,5
Compressive pneumothorax	2	**7,7**
Pericardial tamponade	1	3,8

Thoracotomy approaches		
Postero-laterale	13	**50,0**
Antero-lateral	8	30,8
Median sternotomy	3	11,6
Clamshell	1	3,8
Semi-Clamshell	1	3,8
Gestures		
Lung reminders	18	**69,2**
Costal fixation	9	34,6
Decortication	2	7,7
Pericardial fenestration	1	3,8
Intraoperative pleural drainage		
Two drains	15	57,7
A drain	11	42,3

Pënëtransient trauma accounted for 62% of thoracotomy indications (see Figure 25).

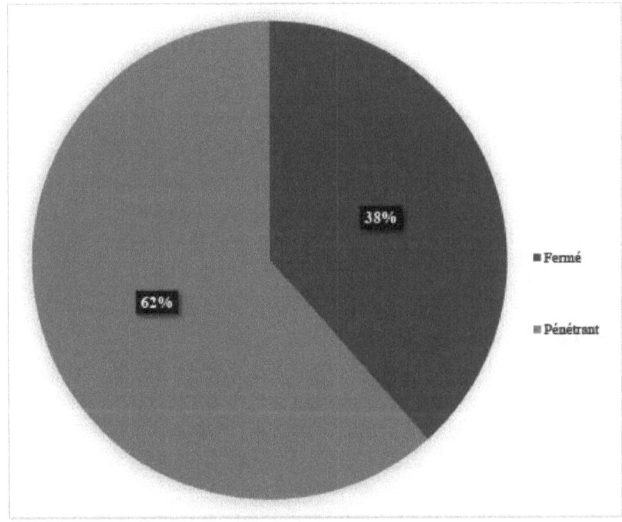

Figure 20: Distribution of thoracotomy indications by type of trauma (n=26)

The median time to pleural drain removal was **4 [2-7]** days, with extremes ranging **from 1** to **34**.

I. Abundant hemothorax (46.4%) was the first indication for pleural drainage (see Table XIV).

Table XIII: Characteristics of pleural drainage

Variables	Numbers (n=46)	Percentages (%)
Drainage methods		
A drain	**67**	**81,7**
Two drains	15	18,3

Types of drainage assembly		
Underwater only	**63**	**76,8**
Vacuum then underwater	12	14,6
Vacuum only	7	8,6
Drainage indications		
Abundant haemothorax	38	**46,4**
Hemopneumothorax	26	31,7
Abundant pneumothorax	18	21,9
Drain insertion sites		
5[eme] intercostal space	60	**73,1**
6[eme] intercostal space	14	17,1
4[eme] intercostal space	8	9,8
Exsufflation	**20**	**5,6**

Non-invasive ventilation (58.6%) was the most frequent mode of ventilation.

The only invasive ventilation modality used was orotracheal intubation.

Table XIV: Characteristics of resuscitation measures

Variables	Numbers (N=358)	Percentages (%)
Vascular filling	82	22,9
Blood transfusion	65	**18,2**
Administration of vasopressor drugs	20	5,6
Administration of cardiotonics	15	4,2
External cardiac massage	5	1,4
Number of patients ventilated	99	**27,7**
Ventilation mode (n=99)		
Non-invasive	58	58,6
Invasive	41	41,4
Type of invasive ventilation (n=41)		
Orotracheal intubation	41	**100**
Traclieotomy	0	0
Ventilation type (=99)		
Spontanee	74	**74,5**
Mecanics	25	25,5

Tramadol (92.3%) was the most frequently used analgesic.

Analgesics were most often started by injection (93.2%).

Table XV: Characteristics of analgesic treatment

Variables	Numbers (N=358)	Percentages (%)
Use of analgesics	352	**98,3**
Type of analgesics (n=352)		
Tramadol	327	**92,3**
Non-stëroid anti-inflammatory	213	60,5
Paracëtamol	210	59,6
№fopam	49	13,9
Morphine	1	0,3

Route of administration (n=352)		
Injectable	**328**	**93,2**
Per os	24	6,8

Incentive kinesitherapy was most often dëbutëed on the first day of hospitalisation (55.1%).

Corticosteroids were administered as prophylaxis in 16.2% of victims (see Table XVII).

Table XVI: Characteristics of prophylactic measures

Variables	Numbers (N=358)	Percentages (%)
Incentive kinesitherapy	**98**	**27,4**
Start date of kinesitherapy in hospital days (n=98)		
Day 1	54	**55,1**
Day 2	28	28,6
Day 3	12	12,3
Day 4	2	2,0
Day 5	2	2,0
Gastric protection	207	**57,8**
Administration of corticosteroids	58	**16,2**
Antibiotic prophylaxis	217	**60,6**

The mëdian duration of hospitalisation was **3 [1-9]** days with extremes ranging from **0** to **100** days.

Complications occurred in 94 patients **(26.3%)**.

Acute respiratory distress syndrome **(43.6%)** ë-was the most common complication.

Table XVII: Distribution of patients according to length of hospitalisation and complications.

Variables	Numbers (N=358)	Percentages (%)
Duration of hospitalisation in days		
[0-5[	**208**	**58,1**
[5-12[	97	27,1
12	53	14,8
Complications	**94**	**26,3**
Nature of complications (n=94)		
ARDS*	**41**	**43,6**
Pneumonia/Empyëme	30	31,9
ACR**	10	10,7
Secondary bleeding	8	8,5
Other	3	3,2
Rëinterventions	2	2,1

ARDS*=Acute Respiratory Distress Syndrome

CHF**=Cardio-Respiratory Arrest

Other***=Arrhythmia, disorders of dëglutition and mëdiastinitis.

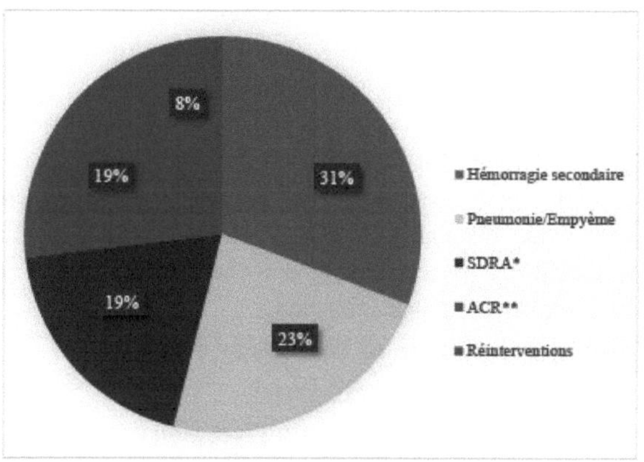

Figure 21. Distribution of post-operative thoracotomy complications (n=26)

Secondary bleeding (31%) was the most frequent complication after thoracotomy (Figure 27).

The overall mortality rate was **13.6%.**

The mortality rate was highest after thoracotomy (38.5%).

Table XVIII: Distribution of patients according to vital prognosis

Variables	Numbers (N=358)	Percentages (%)
Vital prognosis of patients at the end of treatment		
1'hospitalisation (N=358)		
Deaths	**48**	**13,4**
Survival	310	86,6
Mortality by treatment modality		
Thoracotomy (n=26)	10	**38,5**
Medical treatment combined with pleural drainage (n=46)	12	26,0
Medical treatment alone (n=250)	25	10,0

VII- DISCUSSION

Thoracic trauma is the backbone of trauma care worldwide. Their incidence continues to rise, particularly in sub-Saharan Africa. The need to address this issue also lies in their insidious nature, their high potential for harm and the complexity of their management. Twenty years after the study by *Chichom et al* [19] at the Yaounde General Hospital, the general aim of our work was to assess the factors associated with the current management of thoracic trauma at the Yaounde University Hospital (CHUY) and the Yaounde Emergency Centre (CURY). To achieve our objective, we conducted a cross-sectional analytical study with retrospective data collection.

VII.1 Epidemiological profile of the study population

VII.1.1 Socio-demographic characteristics

In our sample (N=358), age ranged from 1 to 96 years with a median of 30 (2340) years, similar to the results reported by *Getachew et al* [53] in Ethiopia and *Massaga et al* [58] in Tanzania. This median was 10 years less than the average found by *Chichom et al* [19] in 2003 at the Yaounde General Hospital. This difference could be explained by the fact that victims under the age of sixteen were not included in their study.

There was a very clear male predominance (82.7%). These results were identical to those shown by *Tomta et al* [59] in Togo and by *Yena et al* [60] in Mali. Many authors suggest that the high frequency of the twenty to forty age group is due to their greater mobility [61].

The informal sector (49.7%) was the main sector of professional activity. This result is in line with the socio-demographic data in the African Development Bank (ADB) report on Cameroon in 2018 [62]. Motorbike accidents

were the most frequent circumstances of occurrence, as noted by *Tomta et al* [59] in Togo. Very few patients (6.4%) had taken out an insurance policy. This could be explained by the presence of four times as many active or retired civil servants in our sample as in the general population [62]. In Greece in 2000, *Sanidas et al* [63] found that 73.6% of civil servants had insurance cover. This state of affairs creates a clear north-south disparity in the quality of patient care.

VII.1.2 Frequency of thoracic trauma by year

The frequency of thoracic trauma (compared with other trauma) in 2016 (13.3%) was identical to that recorded by *Ludwig et al* [18] in Germany. In Ethiopia, *Getachew et al* [53] showed a frequency of 10% in 2016. This tegere diffërence could be explained by the non-inclusion in their ëtude of patients with simple thoracic contusion. The mean overall frequency (16.5%) in our ëtude ël͡эк similar to the mean annual frequencies of recent European sëries [46].

In 2016, the frequency of thoracic trauma ëlэк more ëlevëe at the Centre Hospitalier et Universitaire (CHUY) than at the Centre des Urgences de Yaoundë (CURY). This finding could be Hë to the fact that in 2016, the CURY was only in its firstë year of existence and was still mëknown to the population. All other years, this frequency ëlə11 each time more ëlevëe at CURY than at CHUY. This could be explained by the renovation work underway at CHUY since 2017, which is limiting its capacity to receive patients.

The World Bank's 2020 report on Cameroon over the last twenty years showed a peak in the incidence of road traffic accidents in 2019 [64]. This could therefore justify the peak in the frequency of thoracic trauma in 2019. The decline in frequency between 2019 (24.4%) and 2020 (19.4%) could be due to the occurrence of the SARS-Cov 2 pandemic, which has had the effect of reducing people's mobility and therefore the number of road accidents in 2020.

VII.2 Clinical and paraclinical profiles

VII.2.1 Clinical characteristics

V II.2.2.1 Anamnestic characteristics

The median time to emergency arrival in our study was similar to that shown by *Ogunrombi et al* [65] in Nigëria in 2012.

Road traffic accidents and stabbings were the main causes respectively of pënëtransplant trauma, as in most of the world's sëries [12,46,58]. However, *Yabre et al* [66] in Burkina Faso and *Ali et al* [67] in Nigeria showed that firearm injuries were the leading cause of pënëtrant trauma in their countries. It should be noted that these two West African countries regularly face terrorist attacks and/or the existence of hotbeds of intercommunity conflict in which firearms are often used.

Motorbike accidents (62.3%) were the main cause of traffic accidents. This finding is repeated in most African and Western sëries [13,54,59,60]. Passengers are most often affected, as shown by *Okonta et al* [54] in Nigeria and *Tomta et al* [59] in Togo.

The frequency of comorbidities in our sample was five times higher than that reported by *Lema et al* [68] in Tanzania. It should be noted that certain conditions such as arterial hypertension and chronic smoking, which can worsen the prognosis of thoracic lesions, were not taken into account in their study. However, arterial hypertension was the main comorbidity in our study population.

V II.2.2.2 Primary balance characteristics

The median Revised Trauma Score (RTS) was 7.84 whereas *Lema et al* [68] found a value of 7.61. This discrepancy in figures may be due to the smaller size of their sample (N=150). The frequency of patients in shock (10%) was three times lower than in the study by *Emircan et al* [69] in Turkey. This difference may be due to the fact that, in their study, most patients were taken to emergency within thirty minutes of the incident. However, in our context, most seriously injured victims die at the scene of the accident [19].

V II.2.2.3 Characteristics of thoracic and associated lesions

Firm thoracic trauma was largely predominant, as in many series [13,18,19,58]. However, *Yena et al* [60] in Mali and *Adegboye et al* [70] in Nigeria showed a predominance of penetrating trauma. This difference may be due to the presence of terrorist factions and recurrent intercommunity conflicts in these countries.

Pulmonary contusion (65.4%) was the most frequent thoracic lesion after firm trauma. In the study by *Chichom et al* [19] in Yaounde in 2003, rib fractures predominated. This diffërence could be explained by the fact that our study population ëЬ-яИ much younger than theirs. However, because of the great elasticity of the ribs in the young subject, the younger a person is, the more likely they are to present with a pulmonary contusion rather than a rib fracture [29]. Patients with rib fractures very often had fewer than three fractured ribs, as shown by *Tomta et al* [60] in Togo and *Demirrhan et al* [71] in Turkey. The costal flap (9.8%) had a frequency identical to that found by *Bouchhab et al [72]* in Morocco and double that found by *Okugbo et al* [73] in Nigëria. This diffërence could be explained by the predominance of pë^^ята trauma in their ëtude. I.'liemopneumotliorax (67.5%) ël эк the most frequent thoracic tesion after pënëtrant trauma as reflected by *Chichom et al.* [19] at the Yaoundë General Hospital and *Massaga et al.* [58] in Tanzania. Cranio-encëphalic injuries were the most frequent associated tesions, as in most series, both Western and African [13, 18, 19, 58, 74, 75]. *Chichom et al* [19] found a mëdian Injury Severity Score (16.9) tegereally lower than in our study. This can be explained by the fact that they did not include victims of ballistic trauma. However, these are responsible for very severe tesions [46].

VII.2.2 Paraclinical characteristics

Standard chest X-ray and CT scan had similar frequencies to those shown by *Chichom etal.* [19] at the General Hospital in 2003. Thoracic ultrasound was ël ërarely requested in our ëstudy as noted by *Chichom et al* [19]. In our ëtude, thoracic ultrasound ël эк more effective in the diagnosis of pneumothorax and hemothorax than chest radiography as shown byMcEwan *et al.* after a mëta- analysis [76].

VII.3. Therapeutic management and results

VII.3.1 Payment arrangements

VII.3.1.1 Specific treatment

Medical treatment alone is the most common management modality (69.9%), as found by many authors [18,19,54,60,68]. Our thoracotomy frequency (7.3%) is half that reported by *Chichom et al* [19] at the Yaoundë General Hospital in 2003. This could be explained by the current unavailability of extracorporeal circulation (ECC) in our two study sites, making surgery impossible where it is essential. During their study period, however, it was functional.

Persistent haemorrhage despite medical treatment combined with pleural drainage represented the main indication for thoracotomy as in many sëries [67,70,73]. Thoracotomy by the postëro-latëral ëtomy route was the most frequently practised as noted by *Ali et*

al. [67] in Nigeria. The antero-lateral route was the most frequent in the study by *Anisuzzaman et al* [78] in Bangladesh. According to *Ludwig et al* [18], posterolateral thoracotomy has the advantage of reducing the risk of accidental injury to intra-thoracic organs. However, according to *Heus et al* [79], in the event of trauma to an organ of the anterior mediastinum, antero-lateral thoracotomy should be preferred. In line with the results of *Chichom et al* [19], lung resection was the most frequently performed surgical procedure in our study.

Large hemothorax (46.4%) was the first indication for pleural drainage, as shown by *Chichom et al.* [19] and numerous series [13,14,25,29,58,59,64]. The closed circuit underwater drainage system (77%) was the most widely used, as shown by several studies carried out in conditions similar to ours [58,67,73]. All the patients in whom double drainage was used were those who had undergone thoracotomy, as reported by *Ogunrombi et al* [65] in Nigeria. The drains were usually inserted at the intersection of the fifth intercostal space and the middle axillary line, as reported by *Ngo Nonga et al* [39] in Yaounde and *Ali et al* [67] in Nigeria. According to *Ali et al* [67], the site of chest tube insertion should depend on the nature of the effusion, its density and the patient's position of comfort. Thus, according to the same authors, because of the density of the blood, insertion of the drain in the fourth intercostal space in the case of hemothorax would reduce its effectiveness; on the other hand, placing the drain in the sixth intercostal space if there is an air component in the effusion would also reduce its effectiveness [67].

VII.3.1.2 General measures

We found that a quarter of patients were transfused and the main indication was haemorrhagic shock, as reported by *Okugbo et al* [73] in Nigeria. Half of ventilated patients were ventilated mechanically after orotracheal intubation, as reported by *Chichom et al* [19] in Yaounde in 2003. According to learned societies, morphine, a strong opioid, is the reference analgesic after thoracic trauma. However, it remains financially inaccessible for many patients in our context [19,65,67]. In our study, tramadol (92.3%) was the most prescribed analgesic. This can be explained, on the one hand, by its low cost and availability in our pharmacies and, on the other hand, by the existence of combinations that can alleviate severe pain.

The frequency of incentive kinesitherapy (28%) was similar to that reported by *Yena et al* [60] in Mali. The frequency of patients receiving gastric protection (57.8%) was identical to that reported by *Ali et al* [67] in Nigeria.

VII.3.2 Future developments

We found a median length of hospitalisation identical to that reported by *Anisuzzaman et al* [78] in Bangladesh. This median was two times lower than that reported in several African series [58,65,67]. This could be explained by the presence in our sample of a large number of patients with simple tioracic contusions whose hospital stay rarely exceeded one day

The frequency of complications (26.3%) in our study was similar to that reported in many recent African publications [64,65,72]. However, it was twice as high as that reported by *Chichom et al* [19] in Yaounde in 2003. This dissimilarity may be due to the fact that the median patient severity score (ISS) in our sample was ten points higher than in that of *Chichom et al* [19]. Most of the series carried out both in our context and in the West also found that acute respiratory distress syndrome in adults was the most frequent complication [18]. The nature and frequency of complications following thoracotomy (70%) were identical to those reported in many series in our setting [19,65,67].

The overall mortality rate (13.4%) was half that reported by *Massaga et al* [58] in Tanzania and almost identical to those found in several Western studies [13,46,52,71]. This closeness of the figures to the Western series suggests that the technical platform may be less important in the balance of mortality compared with the experience of the teams.

VII.4. Strengths and limitations of the study

VII.4.1 Study strengths

> тепёе study in two centres
> Large sample size

VII.4.2 Difficulties and limitations of the study

The difficulties and limitations of this ëtude ëtaient principalement ceux des ëtudes retrospectives portant sur les dossiers de patients notamment :

> The archiving system was not numërisë
> Files were often not rangës at archive level
> The files were often difficult to use because of their condition.
> Information about trauma and antëcëdents was often not dëtaillës.
> The oldest emergency registers ëwere sometimes impossible to find.

VIII-CONCLUSION

Thoracic trauma tends to affect young male adults. Victims generally present to emergency with a firm trauma. Road traffic accidents are the leading cause. Pulmonary contusion is the most common lesion. Thoracic trauma commonly presents with associated lesions. Cranioencephalic trauma is the main extra-thoracic site. Chest X-rays are almost always performed, and ultrasound is rarely used. Conservative treatment combined with thoracic drainage is the mainstay of management. Thoracotomy is rare. It is usually performed after penetrating trauma. The posterolateral approach is predominant. Thoracic drainage is usually underwater and is usually effective in treating large or mixed pleural effusions. Complications are frequent, the main one being acute respiratory distress syndrome in adults. Most patients spend less than five days in hospital. The overall mortality rate is low and patients usually die following thoracotomy.

IX- RECOMMENDATIONS

We humbly submit these demands.

> **To the Ministry of Public Health :**

- Equip the emergency departments of all hospitals from level III upwards with a free kit for immediate care (analgesics, intubation equipment, cardiac resuscitation drugs, pleural drains).
- Provide intensive care units with more respirators and oxygen cylinders.
- Extend universal health insurance, even partially, to patients in a state of absolute vital emergency.

> To the **Deans of Cameroon's Faculties of Medicine:**

- Increase the number of hours devoted to lectures and practical work on the most common emergencies.

> To the **Directors of CHUY and CURY :**

- Computerising the archiving of patient data
- Regularly hold practical workshops on the ABCDEs

> To **care teams:**

- Request a ëpleural ultrasound in a patient with suspected post-traumatic pleural effusion prior to pleural drainage.
- Starting resuscitation measures on admission would reduce the number of thoracotomies and complications.
- Counsel all adult patients about the dangers of speeding.

> To the **general population**:

- Respect the rules of road safety because road accidents can be very serious.

fatal, particularly as a result of trauma to the thorax.

- Avoid driving a vehicle while under the influence of alcohol

X- BIBLIOGRAPHICAL REFERENCES

1. Baker SP, O'Neill R, Karpf RS. The Injury Fact Book. Lexington, Mass: Lexington Books, 1984.

2. Butcher NE, D'Este C, Balogh ZJ. The quest for a universal definition of polytrauma: A trauma registry-based validation study. Jr Trau. Acute Care Surg, 2014, 77 (4): 620-3.

3. Karmy-Jones R, Jurkovich G. Blunt Chest Trauma. Curr. Probl. Surg, 2004, 41:223-380.

4. Ciesla D, Moore E, Johnson J, Burch J, Cothren C, Sauaia A. The role of the lung in postinjury multiple organ failure, Surgery 2005, 138:749-58.

5. Murray JL, Lopez AD. A comprehensive assessment of mortality and disability from diseases, injuries, and risk factors in 1990 and projected to 2020. Har. School Pub. Hea (WHO), 1996.

6. Sauaia A, Moore F, Moore E, Moser K, Brennan R, Read R, et al. Epidemiology of trauma deaths: a reassessment. Jr Trau, 1995, 38:185-93.

7. McQueen KA, Hagberg C, McCunn M. The Global Trauma Burden and Anesthesia Needs in Low- and Middle-Income Countries. Am. Soc Anes, 2014, 78(6):16-19.

8. Nantulya VM, Reich MR. The neglected epidemic: road traffic injuries in developing countries. Br. Med. Jr, 2002, 324:1139-41.

9. Clark GC, Schecter WP, Trunkey DD. Variables affecting outcome in blunt chest trauma: Flail chest vs. pulmonary contusion. Jr Trau 1988; 28:298-304.

10. World Health Organization. Global burden of disease: 2004 update. 2008.

11. Chichom-Mefire A, Mbarga-Essim T, Monono EM, Ngowe M. Compliance of District Hospitals in the Center Region of Cameroon with WHO/IATSIC Guidelines for the Care of the injured: A Cross-Sectional Analysis. World Jr Surg, 2014, 38:2525-33.

12. Balock JB, Ochsner JL. Management of thoracic trauma. Surg. Clin. Nor. Am, 1996, 46(6).1513-24.

13. Kulshrestha P, Munshi I, Wait R. Profile of chest trauma in a level I trauma center. Jr Trau, 2004, 57:576-81.

14. Stewart MR, Rotondo FM, Henry SM, Drago M, Merrick C, Haskin DS et al. International Awg. Advanced trauma life support (ATLS(R)): the ninth edition. Jr. Trau. Ac. Ca. Su. 2013, 74:1363-6.

15. McGreevy J, Stevens KA, Monono EM, Mballa GA, Ngamby KM, Hyder AA et al. Road traffic injuries in Yaoundë, Cameroon: A hospital-based pilot surveillance study. Int. Jr. Care Inj, 2014, 45(2014):1687-92.

16. Waydhas C. Thoracic trauma. Unfallchirurgie, 2000, 103:871-89.

17. Kesieme EB, Ocheli EF, Kesieme CN, Kaduru CP. Profile of thoracic trauma in two semi urban university hospitals in Nigeria. Prof. Med. Jr, 2011, 18(3):373-9.

18. Ludwig C, Koryllos A. Management of chest trauma. Jr. Th. Dis. 2017; 9(3):172-7.

19. Chichom-Mefire A, Pagbe JJ, Fokou M, Ngimbous JF, Guifo ML, Bahebeck J. Analysis of epidemiology, lesions, treatment, and outcome of 354 consecutive cases of blunt and penetrating trauma to the chest in Africa setting. Sou. Afr. Jr Sci, 2010, 48(3):90-3.

20. Abenojo SA. Management of chest trauma: a review. West. Afr. Jr, 1993, 12(2):122-

32.
21. Solagberu BA, Adekanye AO, Ofoebgu CP, Udofia US, Abdur-Rahman LO, Taiwo JO. Epidemiology of trauma deaths. West Afr. Jr Med 2003; 22(2):177-81.
22. Roberts KP, Weinhaus AJ. Anatomy of the Thoracic Wall, Pulmonary Cavities, and Mediastinum. Handbook of Cardiac Anatomy, Physiology, and Devices. Springer, Cham, 2015, p35-60.
23. Netter FK. Atlas of human anatomy. Masson, 3rd ed, p180-8.
24. West JB. Respiratory physiology. 6th ëdition. Paris, Maloine, 2003, p. 222.
25. Avaro JP, Bonnet PM. Management of fermës trauma of the thorax. Rev. Mal. Res. 2011; 28:152-63.
26. Jonsson A, Arvebo E, Schantz B. Intrathoracic pressure variations in an anthropomorphic dummy exposed to air blast, blunt impact and missiles. Jr Trau, 1988, 28(1):125-31.
27. Haberer J. Biomëcanique des traumatismes fermës. In: Beydon, L, Carli, P and Riou. Arnette, Paris, 2000, p27-37.
28. Liden E, Berlin R, Janzon B, Schantz B, Seeman T. Some observations relating to behind- body armour blunt chest trauma caused by ballistic impact. Jr Trau, 1988, 28:145-8.
29. Michelet P, Couret D. Thoracic trauma. Ann. Fr. Ane. Rëa., 2010.
30. Richardson JD, McElvein RB, Trinkle JK. First rib fracture: a hallmark of severe trauma. Ann. Surg, 1975, 181(3):251-4.
31. Woodring JH, Fried AM, Hatfield DR, Stevens RK, Todd EP. Fractures of first and second ribs: predictive value for arterial and bronchial injury. Am. Jr. Ro. 1982; 138(2):211-5.
32. IBique P, Serre T, Cheynel N, Arnoux P, Thollon L, Behr M et al. An experimental cadaveric study for a better understanding of blunt traumatic aortic rupture. Jr Trau, 2006, 61(3):586-91.
33. Von Garrel T, Ince A, Junge A, Schnabel M, Bahrs C. The sternal fracture: radiographic analysis of 200 fractures with special reference to concomitant injuries. Jr Trau, 2004, 57(4):837-44.
34. Rubikas R. Diaphragmatic injuries. Eur. Jr. Card. Surg, 2001, 20(1):53-7.
35. Miller KS, Sahn SA. Chest Tubes: indications, technique, management and complications. Chest, 1987, 91(2):258-64.
36. Eren S, Kantarci M, Okur A. Imaging of diaphragmatic rupture after trauma. Clin Rad, 2006, 61(6):467-77.
37. Zieleskiewicz L, Arbelot C, Hammad E, Brun C, Textoris J, Martin C et al. Lung ultrasound: clinical applications and perspectives in intensive care unit. Ann. Fr. An. Rea, 2012, 31(10):793-801.
38. Leone M, Albanese J, Rousseau S, Antonini F, Dubuc M, Alliez B et al. Pulmonary contusion in severe head trauma patients: impact on gas exchange and outcome. Chest, 2003, 124:2261-6.
39. Ngo-Nonga B, Jemea B, Mouafo TF, Kamgaing N, Bahebeck J, Sosso M. Feasibility of a simple drainage system in Cameroonian children after thoracotomy and decortication for empyema thoracis. Afr. Jr. Paed. Surg, 2012, 9(1):27-31.

40. Bertrand S, Cuny S, Petit P, Trosseille X, Page Y, Guillemot H et al. Traumatic rupture of thoracic aorta in real-world motor vehicle crashes. Traf. Inj. Prev, 2008, 9(2):153-61.
41. O'Conor CE. Diagnosing traumatic rupture of the thoracic aorta in the emergency department. Emerg. Med. Jr, 2004, 21:414-9.
42. Wicky S, Capasso P, Meuli R, Fischer A, von Segesser L, Schnyder P. Spiral CT aortography: an efficient technique for the diagnosis of traumatic aortic injury. Eur. Rad, 1998, 8:828-33.
43. Johnson SB. Tracheobronchial injury. Sem. Thor. Card. Surg. 2008; 20:52-7.
44. Asensio JA, Chahwan S, Forno W, MacKersie R, Wall M, Lake J et al. Penetrating esophageal injuries: multicenter study of the American Association for the Surgery of Trauma. Jr Trau, 2001, 50:289-96.
45. Young CA, Menias CO, Bhalla S, Prasad SR. CT features of esophageal emergencies. Radiographics, 2008, 28:1541-53.
46. Freixinet GF, Rodriguez HH, Vallina PM, Balsalobre RM, Pedro Rodriguez Suarez PR. Guidelines for the Diagnosis and Treatment of Thoracic Trauma. Arch. Bronco, 2011, 47(1):41-9.
47. Rashid MA, Wikstrom T, Ortenwall P. Outcome of lung trauma. Eur. Jr Surg, 2000, 166(6):22-8.
48. Rapsang AG, Shyam DC. Scoring Systems of severity in Patients with Multiple Trauma. Cir. Esp. 2015; 93(4):213-21.
49. Ranieri VM, Rubenfeld GD, Thompson BT, Ferguson ND, Caldwell E, Fan E et al. Acute respiratory distress syndrome: the Berlin Definition. Jr. Am. Med. Asso, 2012, 307(23):2526-33.
50. College of Teachers of Neurology. Non-traumatic comas. 2019.
51. Lociciero J, Kenneth LM. Epidemiology of Chest Trauma. Surg. Clin. North. Am, 1989, 69(1):15-9.
52. Segers P, Van Schil P, Jorens P, Van Den Brandt F. Thoracic trauma: an analysis of 187 patients. Acta. Chi. Belg. 2001, 101(6):277-82.
53. Getachew S, Ali E, Tayler-Smith K, Hedt-Gauthier B, Silkondhez W, Abebe A et al. The burden of road traffic injuries in an emergency department in Addis Ababa, Ethiopia. Pub. Act. Hea. 2016; 6(2):66-71.
54. Okonta KE, Ocheli EO. Blunt Chest Injury: epidemiological profile and determinant of mortality. Int. Surg. Jr, 2018, 5(5):1622-7.
55. Zoa O: Trauma of the thorax in CHU emergencies (Abstract in thesis), Faculte de Mëdecine et des Sciences Biomedicales de Yaounde, 2018.
56. Kasiulevicius V, Sapoka V, Filipaviciute R. Sample size calculation in epidemiological studies. Gerontologija, 2006, 7(4):225-31.
57. Vermeulen B, Konstantinidis P. A priori simple thoracic trauma: what is there to be wary of? Rev. Med. Suisse, 2005, 1:1910-3.
58. Massaga FA, Mchembe M. The Pattern and Management of Chest trauma at Muhimbili National Hospital, Dares Salaam. East. Afr. Jr Med, 2010, 15(1):124-9.
59. Tomta K, Ouedraogo N, Ouro-Bangna F, Songne B. Les traumatismes du thorax :aspects epidemiologiques, cliniques et therapeutiques de 320 cas colliges au CHU de

Tokoin. Afr. Jr On, 2005, 7(2).
60. Yena S, Sanogo ZZ, Sangare DD, Keita AD, Coulibaly Y, Ouattara M et al. Les traumatismes thoraciques a l'hopital du point " G ". Mali Med, 2006, 31(1):43-48.
61. Ziegler DW, Agarwal NN. The morbidity and mortality of rib fractures. Jr Trau, 1994, 37:975-9.
62. Doffonsou RA, Nkodia C. African Economic Outlook 2018. African Development Bank Group, 2019.
63. Sanidas E, Kafetzakis A, Valassiadou K, Kassotakis G, Mihalakis J, Drositis J et al. Management of simple thoracic injuries at a Level I trauma centre: can primary health care system take over? Int. Care Inj, 2000, 31(2000):669-75.
64. World Bank. Mortality caused by road traffic injury is estimated road traffic fatal injury deaths per 100,000 population. 2020.
65. Ogunrombi AB, Onakpoya UU, Ekrikpo U, Adesunkanmi AK, Adejare IE. The Pattern and Outcome of Chest Injuries in South West Nigeria. An. Afr. Surg, 2012, 9(2):78-83.
66. Yabre N, Binyom P, Zare C, Belemliliga LH, Kc'ita N, Sanon G et al. Prise en charge des traumatismes ballistiques du thorax: Un challenge pour une ëquipe chirurgicale de rëfërence de Bobo-Dioulasso. Cahiers CBRSI, Biblio. Nat. Бёши, 2020, 4(18):40-52.
67. Ali N, Gali M. Pattern and Management of Chest injuries in Maiduguri, Nigeria. An. Afr. Med, 2004, 3(4):181-4.
68. Lema MK, Chalya PL, Mabula JB, Mahalu W. Pattern and outcome of chest injuries at Bugando Medical Centre in Northwestern Tanzania. Jr. Cardiothor. Surg, 2011, 6:1-7.
69. Emircan S, Ozgug H, Akkose As, Ozdemir F, Koksal O, Bulut M. Factors affecting mortality in patients of thorax trauma. Turkish. Jr. Tr. Em. Surg. 2011, 17 (4):329-33.
70. Adegboye VO, Ladipo JK, Brimmo IA, Adebo AO. Penetrating chest injuries in civilian practice. Afr. Jr. Med. Sci. 2001; 30(4): 327-31.
71. Demirrhan R, Onan B, Oz K, Halezeroglu S. Comprehensive analysis of 4205 patients with chest trauma: a 10-year experience. Int. Cardiovasc. Thor. Surg. 2009; 9:450-3.
72. Boucchab W, Finech B. Thoracic trauma (thesis), НкиИё de Mëdecine et de Pharmacie de Marrakech, 2009.
73. Okugbo SU, Okoro E, Irhibogbe PE. Chest Trauma in a Regional Trauma Centre. Jr. West. Afr. Coll. Surg, 2012, 2(2): 74-84.
74. Nordberg E. Injuries as a public health problem in sub-Saharan Africa: epidemiology and prospects for control. Ea. Afr. Med. Jr, 2000, 77:1-43.
75. Veysi T, Vassiolis S, Paliobeis NC, Nicolas Efstathopoulos N, Peter Giannoudis P. Prevalence of chest trauma, associated injuries and mortality: a level I trauma centre experience. Int. Ortho, 2009, 33:1425-33.
76. McEwan K, Thompson P. Ultrasound to detect haemothorax after chest injury. Emerg. Med. Jr, 2007, 24(8): 581-2.
77. Seamon MJ, Haut ER, Van Arendonk K, Barbosa RR, Chiu WC et al. An evidence-based approach to patient selection for emergency department thoracotomy: A practice management guideline from the Eastern association for the surgery of trauma. Jr. Trau. Care Surg, 2015, 79(1):159-73.

78. Anisuzzaman, Hosain SN, Reza M, Kibria G, Ferdous S. Management of Chest Trauma in Bangladesh Perspective: Experience of a Decade. Cardiovasc. Jr, 2019, 12(1): 3-8.

XI-ANNEXES

Appendix 1: Ethical clarity

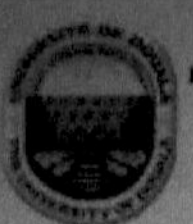

REPUBLIQUE DU CAMEROUN
Paix - Travail- Patrie
•
UNIVERSITE DE DOUALA

REPUBLIC OF CAMEROON
Peace - Work- Fatherland
•
UNIVERSITY OF DOUALA

CEI - UD

INSTITUTIONAL ETHICS COMMITTEE FOR RESEARCH ON HUMAN HEALTH

N°2883 CEI-UDo/07/2021/T

Douala, le 21 Juillet 2021

CLAIRANCE ÉTHIQUE

Le Comité d'Ethique Institutionnel de la Recherche pour la Santé Humaine de l'Université de Douala (CEI-UDo) en sa session du 21 Juillet 2021, a examiné le projet de recherche intitulé **«Prise en charge des traumatismes thoraciques de 2016 à 2020: cas du Centre Hospitalier et Universitaire de Yaoundé et du Centre des Urgences de Yaoundé»** soumis par **MBOUNA MASSIN Stéphane Fargeon**, tenant lieu de Thèse à l'Institut Supérieur de Technologie Médicale (ISTM).

Le présent projet de recherche est d'un intérêt scientifique certain et ne présente aucun risque pour le participant. Les objectifs et la méthodologie de l'étude sont clairement décrits. Le principe de confidentialité des données est respecté. Les compétences requises pour la supervision des travaux de recherche sont présentes.

Au vu de ce qui précède, le CEI-UDo approuve pour une durée d'un an, la mise en œuvre de la présente version du protocole.

MBOUNA MASSIN Stéphane Fargeon est responsable du respect scrupuleux du protocole et ne devrait y apporter aucun amendement aussi mineur soit-il, sans avis favorable du CEI-UDo. Les investigateurs sont tenus de collaborer avec le CEI-UDo pour le suivi des aspects éthiques du protocole approuvé. Le rapport final du projet de recherche devra être déposé au CEI-UDo pour archivage.

La présente clairance éthique est délivrée pour servir et valoir ce que de droit. Elle peut être annulée en cas de non-respect de la réglementation en vigueur et des recommandations sus-mentionnées.

Ampliations
- MINSANTE

LE PRESIDENT

CEI-UD

Pr Léopold Gustave LEHMAN

NB : Il n'est délivré qu'un seul exemplaire de la clairance éthique.

N° 0977/Minsante/SESP/SG/DROS of April 16, 2012
Campus de Logbessou, 3è étage du bloc pédagogique de la FMSP.
Tél. : (237) 680.35.98.35 / 695.39.35.50 / B.P. : 2701 Douala - Cameroun / e-mail : cei@univ-douala.com

Appendix 3: Research authorisation Centre Hospitalier et Universitaire de Yaounde (CHUY)

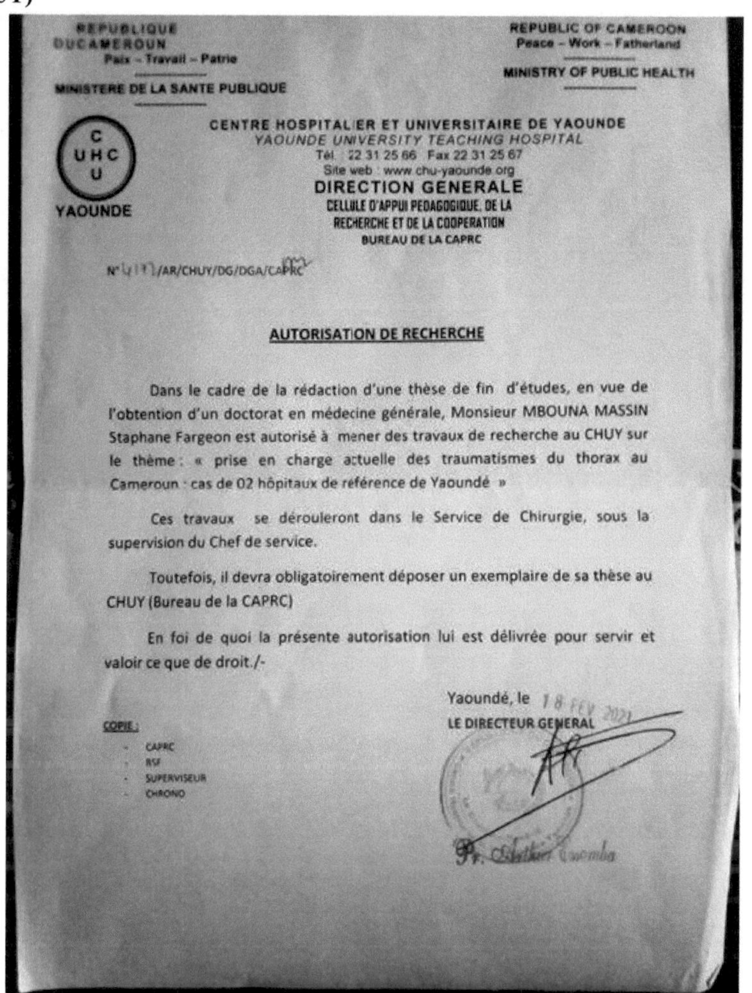

REPUBLIQUE DU CAMEROUN
Paix – Travail – Patrie

MINISTERE DE LA SANTE PUBLIQUE

REPUBLIC OF CAMEROON
Peace – Work – Fatherland

MINISTRY OF PUBLIC HEALTH

CUHCU YAOUNDE

CENTRE HOSPITALIER ET UNIVERSITAIRE DE YAOUNDE
YAOUNDE UNIVERSITY TEACHING HOSPITAL
Tél. : 22 31 25 66 Fax 22 31 25 67
Site web : www.chu-yaounde.org
DIRECTION GENERALE
CELLULE D'APPUI PEDAGOGIQUE, DE LA RECHERCHE ET DE LA COOPERATION
BUREAU DE LA CAPRC

N° 417 /AR/CHUY/DG/DGA/CAPRC

AUTORISATION DE RECHERCHE

Dans le cadre de la rédaction d'une thèse de fin d'études, en vue de l'obtention d'un doctorat en médecine générale, Monsieur MBOUNA MASSIN Staphane Fargeon est autorisé à mener des travaux de recherche au CHUY sur le thème : « prise en charge actuelle des traumatismes du thorax au Cameroun : cas de 02 hôpitaux de référence de Yaoundé »

Ces travaux se dérouleront dans le Service de Chirurgie, sous la supervision du Chef de service.

Toutefois, il devra obligatoirement déposer un exemplaire de sa thèse au CHUY (Bureau de la CAPRC)

En foi de quoi la présente autorisation lui est délivrée pour servir et valoir ce que de droit./-

Yaoundé, le 18 FEV 2021
LE DIRECTEUR GENERAL

COPIE :
- CAPRC
- RSF
- SUPERVISEUR
- CHRONO

Appendix 3: Research authorisation Yaounde Emergency Centre (CURY)

REPUBLIQUE DU CAMEROUN
Paix-Travail-Patrie

MINISTERE DE LA SANTE PUBLIQUE

SECRETARIAT GENERAL

CENTRE DES URGENCES DE YAOUNDE

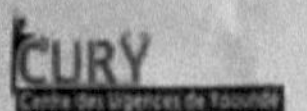

REPUBLIC OF CAMEROON
Peace-Work-Fatherland

MINISTRY OF PUBLIC HEALTH

SECRETARIAT GENERAL

YAOUNDE EMERGENCY CENTER

BP : 3911
E-mail : cury.minsante@Yahoo.fr
Tél : 222 22 25 25/222 22 25 24/222 22 25 22
N° 02104 /A/MINSANTE/SG/DCURY

Yaoundé, le 3 1 MARS 2021

AUTORISATION DE RECRUTEMENT

****

Je soussigné **Dr Louis Joss BITANG à MAFOK**, Directeur du Centre des Urgences de Yaoundé,

Autorise, **Monsieur MBOUNA MASSIN Stéphane Fargeon, Résident de chirurgie général**, étudiant de 7ème année à l'Institut supérieur de technologie médicale de Nkolodom-Yaoundé, de mener un recrutement des malades dans notre Institution Hospitalière pour son mémoire placé sous le thème « ***prise en charge actuelle des traumatismes du thorax au Cameroun : cas du Centre Hospitalier et Universitaire de Yaoundé et du Centre des Urgences De Yaoundé*** », sous la supervision du Dr BITANG à MAFOK Louis Joss.

En foi de quoi la présente autorisation lui est délivrée pour servir et faire valoir ce que de droit./-

Le Directeur

Dr. Louis Joss BITANG à MAFOK
Chirurgien
Directeur du Centre des Urgences de Yaoundé (CURY)

Appendix 4: Data sheet

N°	Question	YearCode	Answer
SECTION I: SOCIO-DEMOGRAPHIC CHARACTERISTICS			
S1Q1	**Age (in years)**		
S1Q2	**Gender**	1=Male2=Female	
S1Q3	**Profession**		
S1Q4	**Insured patient?**	1=Yes2=No	
S1Q5	**Level of education**	1=Never frequented2=Primary 3=Secondary4=University	
S1Q6	**Incident location**		
SECTION II: ANAMNESTIC DATA			
S2Q1	**Patient refere ?**	1=Yes2=No	
S2Q2	**Incident-arrival time (hr)**		
S2Q3	**Means of transport**	1=Mëdicalisë2=No mëdicalisë	
S2Q4	**Cause of trauma**	1=Traffic accident 2=Fall3=Aggression/riot 4=Suicide attempt 5=Other	
S2Q5	**If other, please specify**		
S2Q6	**What type of MVA?**	1=Vëhicle-Piëton 2=Vëhicle-Vëhicle 3 Single vehicle	
S2Q7	**If vehicle-pieton, patient is**	1=Driver 2=Passenger 3=Pieton	
S2Q8	**If vehicle-to-vehicle, patient**	1=Driver 2=Passenger	
S2Q9	**Lesion mechanism**	1=Acceierati on-deceierati on 2=Compression 3=White weapon 4= Firearm 5=Inhalation of foreign bodies 6=Other	
S2Q10	**If other, please specify**		
S2Q11	**If knife, what type?**		
S2Q12	**If foreign body, nature?**		
S2Q13	**Comorbidity**	1=Yes2=No	
If so, which ones?			
S2Q14	**Diabetes**	1=Yes2=No	
S2Q15	**Respiratory insufficiency chronicle**	1=Yes2=No	
S2Q16	**Smoking**	1=Yes2=No	
S2Q17	**Chronic kidney disease**	1=Yes2=No	
S2Q18	**Hepatocellular failure**	1=Yes2=No	
S2Q19	**Heart failure**	1=Yes2=No	

S2Q20	**Pregnancy**	1=Yes2=No	
S2Q21	**If other, please specify**		
SECTION III: CLINICAL DATA			
A: Primary balance			
S3Q1	**VAS status**	1=Free2 Obstructed	
S3Q2	**Frequency respi (cpm)**		
S3Q3	**Heart rate (bpm)**		
S3Q4	**Systolic BP (mmHg)**		
S3Q5	**Glasgow score**		
S3Q6	**SpO2 (%)**		
S3Q7	**Revised Trauma Score**		
B: Lesion assessment			
S3Q8	**Thoracic lesion**	1=LCsion unique2=LCsion multiplc	
S3Q9	**Nature of suspected lesion(s)**	1=Pneumothorax 2=HCmothorax 3=Thoracic laceration 4=Chest contusion 5=Emphysema s/c 6=Rot fracture 7=Costal flap 8=Pulmonary contusion 9=Sternal fracture 10=Diaphragm rupture 11=Bronchial lesion 12=Trachial lesion 13=Aortic rupture 14=Cardiac lesion 15=Resophageal lesion 16=Other	
S3Q10	**If other, please specify**		
S3Q11	**Type of trauma**	1=FermC 2=PCnCtrant	
S3Q12	**Associated lesions**	1=Yes2=No	
If yes, specify number, site of associated lesion(s) and ISS score			
S3Q13	**Number**		
S3Q14	**Site(s)**	1=CranioencCphalic2=Face 3=Knee4=Abdomen 5=Rachis 6=Upper member 7=Lower member 8=Superficial	
S3Q15	**ISS score**		
SECTION IV: PARACLINICAL DATA			
A: Morphological assessment			
S4Q1	**Chest X-ray**	1=Yes2=No	
S4Q2	**Sioui , Lesion(s) retrouvé(s)**	*Use the injury codes above*	
S4Q9	**Chest scan**	1=Yes2=No	
S4Q10	**Sioui , Lesion(s) retrouvé(s)**	*Use the injury codes above*	
S4Q13	**Thoracic ultrasound**	1=Yes2=No	

S4Q14	**Sioui , Lesion(s) retrouvé(s)**	*Use the injury codes above*	
S4Q15	**If other, please specify**		
S4Q16	**Performed in FAST mode**	1=Yes2=No	
S4Q17	**Bronchoscopy**	1=Yes2=No	
B: Biological tests			
S4Q18	**NFS**	1=Yes2=No	
S4Q20	**Creatininemia**	1=Yes2=No	
SECTION V: DONATION THERAPEUTICAL INEES			
S5Q1	**Starting time Specific treatment for lesions (hr)**		
A: Resuscitation			
S5Q2	**Filling**	1=Yes2=No	
S5Q3	**Ventilation**	1=Yes2=No	
S5Q4	**If yes, ventilation mode**	1=Non-invasive2=Invasive	
S5Q5	**If non-invasive ventilation, type of interface**	1=Nose mask 2=Face mask 3=Helmet 4=Goggles 5=Ball	
S5Q6	**Siventilation , mode intubation**	1 Orotraclieale 2 Traclic'otomie	
S5Q7	**Oxygen therapy**	1=Yes2=No	
S5Q8	**SiOxygenotherapie , duration ?**		
S5Q9	**External cardiac massage**	1=Yes2=No	
S5Q10	**Vasopressors**	1=Yes2=No	
S5Q11	**Heart tonics**	1=Yes2=No	
S5Q12	**Blood transfusion**	1=Yes2=No	
B: Pain relief and corticosteroids			
S5Q13	**Analgesics used at start of PEC**	1=Paracetamol2=Nefopam 3=NSAIDs 4=Tramadol 5=Morphine 6=Other	
S5Q18	**Corticotherapy**	1=Yes2=No	
C: Prophylaxis			
S5Q20	**Antibiotic prophylaxis, done?**	1=Yes2=No	
S5Q21	**If so, which TBA?**	1=C3G2=Peni A 3=Quinolone 4=Macrolide 5=Antianaerobes 6=Aminoside 7=Glycopep 8= Peni M	
S5Q22	**Gas protection**	1=Yes2=No	
D : Respiratory kinesitherapy			
S5Q23	**Done?**	1=Yes2=No	
S5Q24	**If yes, date of start of kine**		

E: Specific management of thoracic lesions			
S5Q25	**Curator**	1=Yes2=No	
S5Q26	**Surgical**	1=Yes2=No	
S5Q27	**Type of surgery**	1=Thoracotomy 2=Osteosynthesis 3=Other	
S5Q28	**If other, which?**		
S5Q29	**If thoracotomy, which approach**	1=Postëterior 2=Previous 3=Sternotomy mëdian 4=Clamshell 5=Semi Clamshell 6=Non documentë	
S5Q30	**If surgery, method of anaesthesia**	1=Local 2=Locoregional 3=Gënëral	
S5Q31	**Chest drainage**	1=Yes2=No	
S5Q32	**If drainage, type of drain**	1=Underwater2=Aspirational	
S5Q33	**If DT, time to ablation**		
S5Q34	**Exsufflation**	1=Yes2=No	
SECTION VI: DEVELOPMENT AND PROGNOSIS			
S6Q1	**Length of stay**		
S6Q2	**Complication**	1=Yes2=No	
S6Q3	**If so, which one?**		
S6Q4	**If so, what treatment?**		
S6Q5	**Survival at the end of 1 hospi?**	1=Yes2=No	

Appendix 5: Informed consent form

Appendix 5.1: Informed consent form (in French)

INFORMED CONSENT FORM

Theme: Management of chest trauma in Cameroon: the case of the Yaoundë University Hospital Centre (CHUY) and the Yaoundë Emergency Centre (CURY).

I, the undersigned, Mr/Mrs/Ms, freely accept and agree to voluntarily to participate in the research study entitled "Management of thoracic trauma from 2016 to 2020: Case of the University Hospital Centre of Yaoundë (CHUY) and the Emergency Centre of Yaoundë (CURY)", whose principal investigator is Mbouna Massin Stephane Fargeon under the conditions prëcisëes in the information sheet. I fully understood the information sheet I was given about this ëstudy or else the information sheet relating to this study was read to me and explained. I received all the answers to the questions I asked. The benefits were presented to me and explained. The investigator has made it clear that my participation is free of charge and that I have the right to withdraw from the study at any time. I give my consent for the data collected during this study to be used in subsequent studies or scientific publications.

Done at On

Signature

Appendix 5.2 : Informed consent form (English version)

CONSENT FORM

Theme: Actual management of chest trauma in Cameroon: Case of University Teaching Hospital and Emergency Centre of Yaoundë.

I sub sign Mr, Mrs, Miss freelyand

voluntarily consent in the active participation of my child for the research study entitled "Management of chest trauma from 2016 to 2020: Case of University Teaching Hospital and Emergency Centre of Yaoundë" with Mbouna Massin Stephane Fargeon as main investigator following the precise conditions on the information sheet. I have understood the information notice handed to me concerning this study or I have read and explained the information sheet in relation to this study. I have received all the answers to my questions. The benefits have been presented and explained. The investigator Stephane MBOUNA has precise the free participation and I have the sole right to retrieve from this research at any moment. I give my consent that the collected data during this study should be used for ulterior studies or scientific publications.

Done atOnthe

Signature

Annex 6: Information leaflet

Annex 6.1: Information leaflet (French version)

INFORMATION SHEET

Dear Sir or Madam.

I am Mbouna Massin Stephane Fargeon, ëtudiant en 7e anпёе de mëdecine a l'Institut Supërieur de Technologie Mëdicale. As part of my doctoral thesis in mëdecine, I am conducting a ëtude on the "Prise en charge des traumatismes thoraciques de 2016 a 2020: Cas du Centre Hospitalier et Universitaire de Yaoundë (CHUY) et du Centre des Urgences de Yaoundë (CURY)". This is a ëlиc!e whose aim is to dëcribe the modalities of management of thoracic trauma at the Yaounde Hospital and University Centre (CHUY) and the Yaounde Emergency Centre (CURY) over the last five years. Chest trauma kills more than 5.5 million people every year, with almost 16,000 deaths every day worldwide, 91% of which occur in Africa. However, few studies have been published on the subject in Cameroon. By taking part in this study, you will enable us to carry out a study that could contribute to drawing up national recommendations for the management of thoracic trauma. There is no cost to you for taking part; it is "**totally free**".

The information obtained will be strictly confidential and used exclusively for scientific purposes. The results will be given to the medical team as we are not replacing the treating team. Thank you for your understanding.

If you have any questions about the study, please contact us at the numbers below:

Principal investigator: Stephane MBOUNA: 690592785

Study supervisors: Pr NGO NONGA Bernadette; Drs. BWELLE Georges and BITANG A MAFOK Louis.

Annex 6.2: Information leaflet (English version)

INFORMATION SHEET

Sir, Madam.

I am Mbouna Massin Stephane Fargeon, a 7th year medical student at the Higher Institute of Medical Technology. As part of my doctoral thesis in medicine, I am conducting a study on "Management of chest trauma in Cameroon: Case of the Yaoundë Hospital and University Center (CHUY) and the Yaoundë Emergency Center (CURY)". This is a study whose aim is to describe the modalities of management of trauma to the thorax at the Yaoundë Teaching Hospital (CHUY) and at the Yaoundë Emergency Center (CURY) over the past five years. . In fact, chest trauma kills more than 5.5 million people each year with nearly 16,000 deaths per day worldwide, of which 91% of these deaths occur in Africa. However, there are hardly any published studies on the subject in Cameroon. By taking part in this study, you will allow us to conduct a study that could help to develop national recommendations for the management of chest trauma. Your participation does not incur any costs on your part, it is "completely free".

The information obtained will be strictly confidential and used exclusively for scientific purposes. The results will be given to the medical team because we are not replacing the treatment team. Thanks for your understanding.

If you have any questions about the study, you can contact us at the numbers below:

Principal investigator: Stephane MBOUNA: 690592785

Study supervisors: Prof. NGO NONGA Bernadette; Drs. BWELLE Georges and BITANG A MAFOK Louis.

Appendix 7: Activity timetable

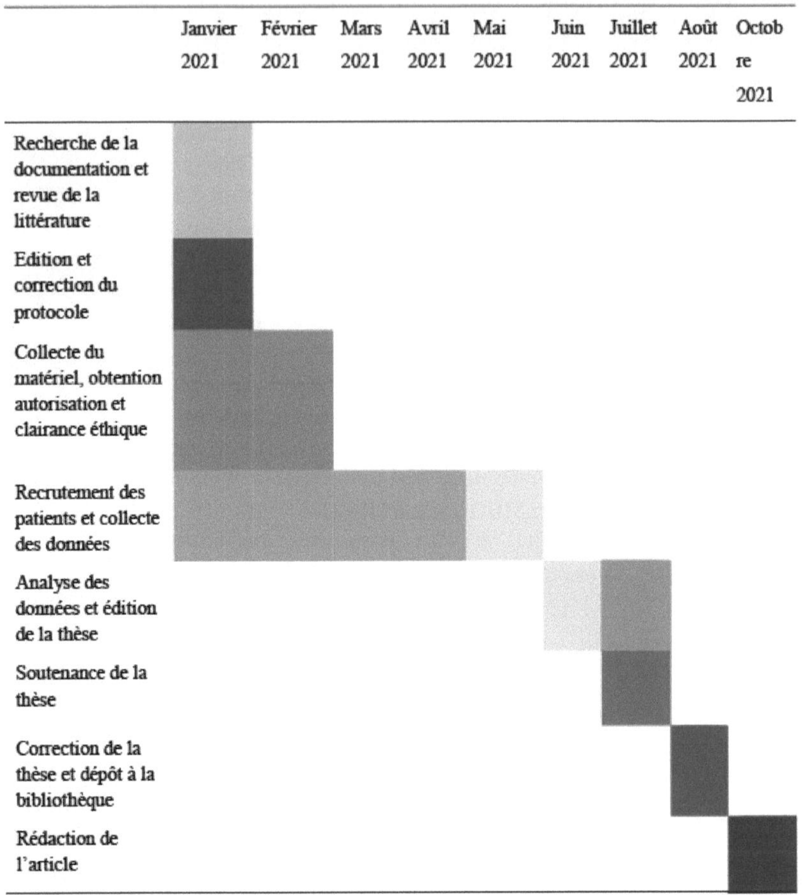

Literature search and review Protocol editing and correction Material collection, authorisation and ethical clearance Patient recruitment and data collection Data analysis and thesis editing Thesis defence Thesis correction and deposit in the library Article writing

Appendix 8: Budgeting

Activities	Object	Cost		
		Unit price (FCFA)	Quantity	Total price (FCFA)
Protocol editing	Documentation	5.000	1	10.000
	Entering and printing	5.000	8	40.000
Carrying out work and collecting data	Technical data	100	200	20.000
	Registers	3.000	3	9.000
	Research authorisations	10. 000	2	20 000
	Teaching materials	/	/	5.000
Data analysis	The statistician's job	50 000	1	50 000
Editing the thesis	Entering and printing the these	5.000	10	50 000
Various	Monthly internet charges	5000	6	30.000
	Transport costs	12.000	6	72.000
Unforeseen	Unforeseen	50.000	/	50.000
TOTAL (FCFA)	/	/	/	356.000
Sources of funding : The family				

Appendix 10: **Severity scores for polytrauma (RTS, AIS and ISS)**

Table I: ***Revised Trauma Score (RTS) [50].***

RTS (Revised trauma score)					
Signs	0	1	2	3	4
Consciousness (Glasgow coma scale)	3	4-5	6-8	9-12	13-15
Systolic blood pressure	0	1-49	50-75	76-89	>89
Respiration rate	0	1-5	6-9	>29	10-29

RTS = 0,9368 (GCS) + 0,7326 (BPs) + 0,2908 (RR)

Minimal score = 0, corresponds to the survival rate = 2,7%.
Maximal score = 7,8408, corresponds to the survival rate = 99%.
The injured patients with the score less than 4 might be transported immediately with the red marking.

The Injury Severity Score ISS is a medical score that used to assess trauma severity and is calculated as follow

1. Read the Abbreviate Injury Scale AIS for six body region i.e. read the AIS from the key board for the "Head ,Face ,Chest, abdomen, extremities and external"
2. Find maximum three AIS
3. Square their value
4. Add them to get ISS

NOTE: AIS rang (0-5) and ISS Should be (0-75)

Write a MATLAB program that used to calculate and display the value of ISS with appropriate message as shown in ISS table below. "Your program should contain at least two user define functions."

ISS calculation Example		
Region	AIS	Max Three Square
Head	0	0
Face	0	0
Chest	4	16
Abdomen	0	0
Extremities	3	9
External	1	1
ISS=16+9+1=26 "Severe "		

ISS Table	
1-8	Minor
9-15	Moderate
16-24	Serious
25-49	Severe
50-74	Critical
75	Maximum

Figure 19: AIS and ISS scores

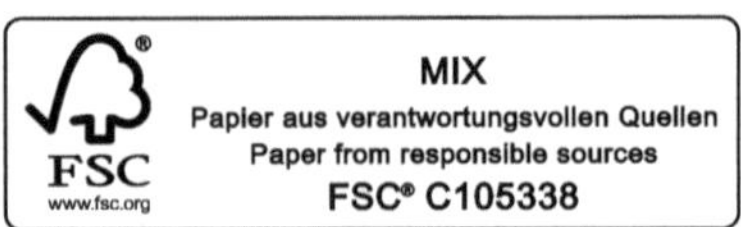

Printed by Books on Demand GmbH, Norderstedt / Germany